EVALUATION IN RURAL COMMUNITIES

Does a program work? What is the value? How do we know? These are questions that keep evaluators up at night. Continued rural community funding, employment, health, and justice depend on our answers to these questions. For evaluators working in rural communities, the task is great, but the return is even greater. Now more than ever before, evaluators have an opportunity to impact social change in rural America.

Beginning with an introduction of rural community evaluation, *Evaluation in Rural Communities* highlights the differences in approaches to evaluation in rural areas, supported by case studies that illustrate key themes and objectives. It explores a number of issues, including

- sustainability
- policy
- cost–benefit analysis
- rural community evaluation as a platform to support social change.

In particular, readers will also learn how to overcome rural community challenges, such as limited resources, the digital divide, limited funding, lower employment and educational attainment, limited opportunities for social interactions, and the distrust of outsiders.

Blending aspects of community-based participatory research, empowerment evaluation, and program evaluation methods, this book is an accessible yet nuanced guide that integrates critical thinking, problem solving, social and political contexts, and outcomes related to evidence-based evaluation.

Allyson Kelley is an Evaluation Scientist with interests in building communities' capacities to address the cultural, social, and environmental factors that contribute differences in health. She has numerous peer-reviewed publications, book chapters, and unpublished evaluation reports that highlight her work in rural America. Her efforts have resulted in the funding and implementation of several successful programs aimed at building the capacity to address disparities using a strength-based approach.

EVALUATION IN RURAL COMMUNITIES

Allyson Kelley

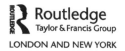
Routledge
Taylor & Francis Group

LONDON AND NEW YORK

First published 2019
by Routledge
2 Park Square, Milton Park, Abingdon, Oxon OX14 4RN

and by Routledge
52 Vanderbilt Avenue, New York, NY 10017

Routledge is an imprint of the Taylor & Francis Group, an informa business

© 2019 Allyson Kelley

British Library Cataloguing-in-Publication Data
A catalogue record for this book is available from the British Library

Library of Congress Cataloging-in-Publication Data
Names: Kelley, Allyson, 1976– author.
Title: Evaluation in rural communities / Allyson Kelley.
Description: 1st Edition. | New York: Routledge, 2019. |
Includes bibliographical references and index.
Identifiers: LCCN 2018035910 | ISBN 9781138312449 (hardback) |
ISBN 9781138312456 (pbk.) | ISBN 9780429458224 (ebook)
Subjects: LCSH: Rural development—Evaluation. | Community
development—Evaluation. | Evaluation research (Social action programs)
Classification: LCC HN49.C6 K43 2019 | DDC 307.1/412—dc23
LC record available at https://lccn.loc.gov/2018035910

ISBN: 978-1-138-31244-9 (hbk)
ISBN: 978-1-138-31245-6 (pbk)
ISBN: 978-0-429-45822-4 (ebk)

Typeset in Bembo
by codeMantra

This book is dedicated to the people who have taught me about evaluation. Program leaders and agency directors, you lead in a way that makes me feel good about what I do and who I am. Evaluation interns and students, your fresh perspective, can-do attitude, and persistence is unmatched. Mentors and teachers, you have shown me a better way to evaluate. Family, friends, and the Creator, thank you.

CONTENTS

List of figures, tables, and boxes   *xii*
Foreword   *xv*
Preface   *xvii*

1 An introduction to evaluation in rural communities   1
   Rural communities 1
   Evaluation 3
   Rural evaluation 4
   Paradigms 4
   Why a text dedicated to rural evaluation? 5
   The rural evaluation process 5
   Implementing, planning, and sustaining rural programs 6
   Summary 7
   Points to remember 7
   Additional reading and resources 8
   Chapter questions 8
   Practice 8
   References 9

2 Context of rural community evaluation   11
   Context and place 11
   Characteristics of rural America 12
   Health 14
   Employment and economy 16
   Poverty 17
   Technology, health care, education, and natural resources 17

Summary 23
Points to remember 23
Additional reading and resources 23
Chapter questions 24
Practice 24
References 25

3 Cultural competence in evaluation 27
What is culture? 27
Understanding the terms 28
Guiding principles for rural evaluators 31
A changing culture 32
Tools for assessing an evaluator's cultural competence 34
Examples of standards that support cultural competence in evaluation 35
Culturally competent resources 37
Case examples with specific cultures in rural America 39
Summary 40
Points to remember 41
Additional reading and resources 41
Chapter questions 41
Practice 42
References 42

4 Evaluation approaches, models, and designs 45
Evaluation approach 45
Evaluation approaches frequently used in rural communities 47
Process and formative evaluation 52
Impact and outcome evaluation 53
Performance monitoring 55
Performance assessment 56
Economic evaluation 56
Evaluation model 59
Evaluation design 61
Research and evaluation 63
Selecting the right approach for rural evaluation 65
Summary 65
Points to remember 65
Additional reading and resources 66
Chapter questions 67
Practice 67
References 67

5 The rural community evaluation process   70
   Planning 70
   Engaging stakeholders and community members 71
   Goals and objectives in the evaluation plan 74
   Identify resources available 76
   Community concerns: the needs of the community 78
   Work plan 79
   Designing the evaluation plan 80
   Theories 82
   Time lines 83
   Data collection plan 83
   Institutional Review Boards 87
   Performance measures and outcomes 87
   Plan for sharing results 88
   Summary 89
   Points to remember 89
   Additional reading and resources 89
   Chapter questions 91
   Activities 91
   References 92

6 How to collect and analyze data in rural communities   93
   Types of data used 93
   Process 93
   Data sources 97
   Quantitative data collection methods 98
   Qualitative data collection methods 99
   Other data collection methods and sources 100
   Data quality 103
   Preparing the data 104
   Data analysis 104
   Analyzing quantitative data 105
   Qualitative data analysis 109
   Mixed methods data analysis 113
   Software 114
   Learnings. Limitations. Assumptions from the data 114
   Summary 115
   Points to remember 115
   Additional reading and resources 115
   Exercises 116
   Activities 117
   References 117

7 Documenting the process, outcome/impact, and economic
program evaluation   120
Formative evaluation 120
Process evaluation 122
Outcome evaluation 123
Impact evaluation 124
Assessment 126
Economic evaluation 127
Summary 129
Points to remember 130
Additional reading and resources 130
Chapter questions 131
Activities 131
References 131

8 Reporting and application of rural evaluation findings   133
Reporting evaluation findings 133
Presenting data 135
Basic elements of an evaluation report 136
Communicating evaluation results 141
Recommendations for applying evaluation findings 142
Best practices for disseminating results 143
Summary 146
Points to remember 147
Additional reading and resources 147
Chapter questions 147
Activities 148
References 148

9 Practical issues for rural evaluators   149
Challenges for rural evaluators from the field 149
Overall challenges from published literature 151
Fit 153
Hiring an evaluator, contracts and agreements 154
Cost of rural evaluation 156
Other cost considerations 156
Opportunities for rural evaluators 157
Education and professional associations 158
Summary 159
Points to remember 159
Additional readings and resources 160

Chapter questions 160
Practice 160
References 161

10 Sustainability and final thoughts for rural evaluators   163
   Sustaining outcomes 163
   What is a sustainability plan? 165
   What factors influence sustainability? 167
   Sustained impacts 168
   Funding future work 169
   Utilizing evaluation for policy change and community transformation 170
   Summary 170
   Final thoughts 170
   Points to remember 171
   Additional readings and resources 171
   Chapter questions 172
   Practice 173
   References 173

Appendix A   Logic Model   175
Appendix B   Evaluation Data Collection   177
Appendix C   Institutional Review Board   178
Appendix D   Forms and Examples   184
Index   191

FIGURES, TABLES, AND BOXES

Figures

2.1	Image USDA Metro and Nonmetro	13
4.1	Logic Model	60
4.2	Prevention Program Outcome Chart	61
4.3	Evaluation Designs	62
4.4	Selecting the Right Evaluation Approach	65
5.1	Five Basic Elements of Rural Evaluation	71
5.2	Steps for Engaging Stakeholders	72
5.3	Developing SMART Goals and Objectives	75
5.4	Field Notes on Rural Community Asset Map for Substance Abuse and Mental Health Services Administration (SAMHSA) Grant	77
5.5	Field Notes on a Rural Program Theory of Change	83
6.1	Thematic Analysis Systems of Care Rural Evaluation	112
6.2	Seven Factors that Determine Validity of Qualitative Data	112
6.3	Field Notes on Triangulating Data	113
8.1	Five-Step Process for Reporting Evaluation Results	134
8.2	Field Notes on Rural Evaluation Reporting with Limited Computer Access	145
8.3	Field Notes on Rural School-Based Recycling Program	145
8.4	Field Notes on Interviews to Document Impact	146
8.5	Field Notes on Documenting Community Perspectives	146
9.1	Evaluation and the Social Determinants of Health in Rural Communities	157
10.1	Factors That Sustain Rural Programs	167
A.1	Rural Waste Program Logic Model	175

A.2 Intervening Variables Logic Model   175
A.3 Rural Prevention Program Logic Model   176
B.1 Data Collection Plan   177
D.1 Needs of Community   188

Tables

2.1 Differences between Rural and Urban Populations   15
2.2 National Rural and Urban Health Comparison   15
3.1 Checklist for Culturally Appropriate Evaluation Methods   34
4.1 Defining Evaluation Purpose, Questions, and Timing   50
4.2 Differences in Research and Evaluation   64
5.1 Active Listening Strategies   74
5.2 Budget Guidelines Example   78
5.3 Field Notes on Identifying Community Concerns in Practice   78
5.4 Field Notes on Goals and Tracking   79
5.5 Field Notes on Outcome Measures in Work Plan   79
5.6 Field Notes on Data in Rural Evaluation   84
5.7 Field Notes on Dissemination Plan   88
6.1 Types of Data   94
6.2 How Data Are Collected   94
6.3 Advantages and Disadvantages of Primary, Secondary, and
      Administrative Data   98
6.4 Field Notes on Evaluative Aims and Analysis Methods   105
6.5 Field Notes on Measures, Frequency Source, Method, and
      Level of Data   105
6.6 Field Notes on Qualitative and Quantitative Software Programs   114
8.1 Active Dissemination Plan   143
8.2 Considering the Best Dissemination Approach for Rural
      Communities   144
9.1 Field Notes on Checklist for Making Sure Evaluators
      Fit Rural Needs   153
10.1 Program Sustainability Framework Domains and Definitions   164
10.2 Field Notes on Sustainability Action Plan   165
10.3 Ten-step Sustainability Plan for Community Coalitions   166
10.4 Field Notes on Funding Strategies, Sources, and Actions   169

Boxes

1.1 Example of a rural solicitation for funding and evaluator's role   6
2.1 Field notes on context   12
2.2 A call for rural-focused evaluation   22
3.1 Field notes on culture and adapting instruments   30
3.2 Field notes, guiding principles for culturally competent evaluation 33

4.1	Impact evaluation formula	53
4.2	Principles of impact evaluation in practice	54
4.3	Considerations for economic evaluations	57
4.4	Field notes on CBA	59
4.5	Field notes on evaluation designs in rural practice	63
5.1	Field notes on trust and credibility	73
5.2	Field notes on evaluation budgets	77
5.3	Field notes on work plans	80
5.4	Field notes on designing an evaluation plan	81
5.5	Field notes on theories	82
5.6	Field notes on data collection	86
6.1	Field notes on evaluation instruments	96
6.2	Probability sampling formula	99
6.3	Field notes on focus groups	100
6.4	Field notes on multiple data sources for meeting funding agency reporting requirements	101
6.5	Rural opioid epidemic web-based news article excerpt	102
6.6	Field notes on instrumentation factors	103
6.7	Field notes on univariate and bivariate outputs	106
6.8	Field notes on qualitative data analysis	111
7.1	Formative evaluation of the healthy corner store initiative	121
7.2	Process evaluation of a promotora de salud intervention	122
7.3	Outcome evaluation of rural head start classrooms	123
7.4	Impact evaluation of the US Department of Education	125
7.5	Participatory assessment of barriers to health care	126
7.6	Economic evaluation of Kentucky Homeplace program	128
7.7	Cost–benefit of bike/pedestrian trails	128
8.1	Field notes on an executive summary	136
8.2	Field notes on evaluation purpose	138
8.3	Field notes on evaluation methods	138
8.4	Field notes on key findings	139
8.5	Field notes on recommendations and lessons learned	140
9.1	Developing a rural citizen engagement plan	153
9.2	Rural program evaluator RFP	154
9.3	External evaluation contract RFP example	155
9.4	Field notes on rural evaluator opportunities	158
10.1	The healthy schools initiative, factors that predict sustainability	168
10.2	Five reasons to evaluate in rural communities	171

FOREWORD

Rural populations have much in common with metropolitan and urban populations. This includes hardworking individuals and families; small and large businesses on the roller coaster of rises and falls of success; unique community and social groups; and a diverse ethnic, racial, and cultural base. However, what make them distinguishable is the degree and extent of the challenges that dramatically affect these commonalities. Given these challenges, programs, services, and levels of accountability for each must be more than just equal to their urban and metro counterparts; they need to be equitable. This means that evaluators working with populations in rural communities must have a clear understanding of the theories of practice, the effective approach, and the unique considerations and characteristics that impact the implementation of a rigorous and targeted assessment effort. This understanding and the "mechanics" of the development and practice of rural community-based evaluation are well laid in this book by Dr. Allyson Kelley.

In Chapter 1, Kelley focuses on a critical aspect of any evaluation effort with vulnerable and complex populations, gaining an appreciation of the unique historical and cultural status of rural communities in the United States. This chapter also introduces the reader to the strengths of the participatory rural evaluation methodology. In Chapter 2, the questions of feasibility and capacity to conduct evaluation with rural communities in consideration of geography, resources, social interactions, community characteristics, political context, and poverty are discussed. Critically, Kelley addresses the key role played by local leaders and government entities involved in programming and evaluation in rural areas. In Chapter 3, the distinctive cultural context of rural communities based on Kelley's own experience and the American Evaluation Association, Guiding Principles for Evaluation are presented. As in the other chapters, Kelley concludes with recommendations for working with culturally diverse populations and provides several resources for practicing culturally competent evaluation. In Chapter 4, Kelley recognizes and explores the reality that there are many participatory evaluation models, approaches, and designs that can be used to meet the needs of programs and services in rural communities. Building on key points covered in the first three chapters, the author walks the evaluator through the crucial decision-making process on the identification and then use of what works best, given the realities of a given project. In Chapters 5 and 6, Kelley walks the reader through the practical and logical best practices for implementing the fundamentals of the rural community evaluation process. Steps, from planning and engaging stakeholders to the design and conduct of the data collection effort to threats to fidelity and their solutions, are covered in specific detail. In Chapters 7 and 8, Kelley argues and provides evidence supporting the thesis that documenting evaluation results is extremely important because it highlights program components, inputs, activities, and outputs through the presentation of various case-based examples of how evaluations are documented based on real-world rural evaluation practice. A key point in this chapter is the recognition that such documentation enhances the reliability and usability of the evaluation effort and its findings to the benefit of rural stakeholders and evaluators wishing to conduct such endeavors. In Chapters 9 and 10, Kelley importantly discusses the issues of replicability of these efforts and the role of evaluators in supporting sustainability planning and evaluation outcomes. These chapters highlight not only opportunities for rural evaluators working in small communities to impact social change and address inequities but also their chance to utilize evaluation findings to fund future work and leveraging of results for future programming, policy development, and guide community capacity building.

In sum, rural communities have unique strengths and provide challenges that must be considered in the evaluation process. Guidance on how best to address these considerations has not been well documented in scholarly texts. Readers will find that Dr. Kelley has not only provided a vibrant and comprehensive undertaking of these considerations but a functional and usable text as well.

Joseph Telfair, DrPH, MSW, MPH
President, American Public Health Association (APHA)
Professor of Public Health Practice and Research, Dual Chair
Department of Community Health
Karl E. Peace Distinguished Chair of Public Health
Jiann-Ping Hsu College of Public Health
Georgia Southern University

PREFACE

I believe that we do not learn evaluation by taking a course or having an advanced degree. I believe that we learn by doing.

This doing has led me to writing this book. I struggled early in my career with translating information presented in a book to use in a rural community. Often, the information did not fit the rural context or culture. Over the years, mentors have shown me how to fit evaluation to the context. Dr. Robert Aronson's work in community-based participatory research served as a model for me to follow. This text supports a community-based participatory approach and the engagement of community members in all phases of the evaluation. Dr. Debra Wallace's leadership in building health equity, Dr. Joseph Telfair's expertise in evaluation methods, Cheryl Belourt's teachings on sovereignty and protocols, and Dr. Dee Big Foot's teachings on trauma-informed methods are the unwritten teachings which this book is based on.

The goal of this book is to guide evaluators, program staff, private organizations, government organizations, educators, students, and community members as they plan and implement evaluations throughout rural America.

Organization of Rural Evaluation

I organized this book based on rural evaluation methods. The first two chapters provide context and information about evaluation in rural America. Chapter 3 describes cultural competence in evaluation and summarizes current tools, standards, and case examples from rural America. Chapter 4 provides an overview of evaluation approaches, models, and designs. Chapter 5 describes the rural community evaluation process from planning to sharing results. Chapter 6 focuses on how to collect and analyze data in rural communities. Chapter 7 uses published evaluations that document results, with a focus on evaluation purpose, questions, timing, and dissemination methods. Chapter 8 provides an overview of how to report and apply rural evaluation findings. Chapter 9 describes practical issues for rural evaluators, along with opportunities for rural evaluators. This book concludes in Chapter 10 with an overview of sustainability and a clear rationale for rural-focused evaluation.

Pedagogical Features

Each chapter begins with a note that I wrote to you, the reader. Throughout the chapters, I use field notes to share evaluation approaches, experiences, and case examples from the field. Each chapter ends with a summary and points to remember. Additional readings and resources are listed for more information on specific topics covered in the chapter. Chapter questions are designed to reinforce topics presented and methods used. Practice questions are included to promote critical thinking, skill building, and knowledge about rural evaluation. References are included at the end of each chapter. The appendix includes examples of logic models, data collection plans, information on Institutional Review Boards, and various evaluation forms.

1

AN INTRODUCTION TO EVALUATION IN RURAL COMMUNITIES

How are rural community evaluations different from those in non-rural communities? This is a question that I asked myself when I started this book. I knew there were differences; I had experienced these differences for more than 10 years, but I never took the time to write them down. This chapter, and this book, is about noticing these differences so that we can be more effective, be more culturally responsive, and evaluate in a more meaningful way.

Rural communities

Rural communities have unique histories, populations, assets, and evaluation needs. With more than 24 definitions of "rural" and various uses for determining the rural classification of geographic regions throughout the United States, it is important to understand these definitions and how we will use them in this book.

In the United States, the federal government uses unique definitions of rural to allocate funding, develop policy, and determine eligibility for special grant programs. There are three federal government programs that have established their own rural definition: the United States Census Bureau, the Office of Management and Budget (OMB), and the Federal Office of Rural Health Policy (FORHP).

- The United States Census Bureau defines rural as any place outside a city or urban cluster with less than 2,500 residents. The Census uses the term rural to include any nonurban population, housing, or territory. Based on the 2010 Census, 59.5 million people or 19.3 percent of the US population was rural, and more than 95 percent of the US land base is considered rural (United States Census, 2017).

- The OMB uses the terms metropolitan, micropolitan, or neither to classify rural areas where metro areas include urban areas of 50,000 people or more and a micro area population is 10,000 people or more but less than 50,000 people. Counties that do not meet the population standards for micro or metro are considered rural. Using the OMB definition of rural, about 46.2 million people in the United States live in rural areas, making up 15% of the total US population and 72% of the land base (Health Resources & Services Administration, 2016).

- The FORHP is another federal government agency with unique definitions of rural. All nonmetro counties (less than 50,000 people) are considered rural by the FORHP. Using Census data to determine county-level designations for rural, FORHP reports that more than 57 million people or 18 percent of the population live in rural America. According to FORHP guidelines, rural American covers 84 percent of the land base (Health Resources & Services Administration, 2016).

In recent years, researchers, policy makers, evaluators, and federal program staff advocated for improving the operational definitions of rural. Recognizing the need to expand dichotomous population views of urban and rural, Harold Goldsmith and colleagues developed a method to more equitably distribute resources and maintain health services in rural communities. The Goldsmith Method uses Census data to identify small towns and rural parts of metro areas in the United States (Goldsmith, Puskin, & Stiles, 2013). For more information on the Goldsmith Method, review the additional resources at the end of this chapter.

A **community** may be defined as a geographic area with boundaries and landmarks (Murphy, 2014) or a group of people with shared interests and characteristics (Eng & Parker, 1994). Communities in rural America have a history that can be traced back to the American Revolution, when more than 90% of the US population lived in rural areas. But industrialization and urbanization changed the face of rural America, and by 1920, the US Census Bureau declared that America was no longer a rural Nation but in fact an urban Nation (Riney-Kehrberg, 2016). During the 1920s, more than 50 percent of the US population lived in towns with more than 2,500 people. Early rural America lacked roads, electricity, running water, and the basic conveniences of an urbanized population. But World War II and the Great Depression changed the face of rural America. With limited access to jobs, education, and food, many people left rural America for refuge in larger towns and cities throughout the United States. Today, the population of rural America continues to decline as people seek modern conveniences and the amenities of urban life. Other factors related to population decline include fewer births than deaths and net migration. From 2010 to 2016, the rural population declined by more than 200,000 people or 0.07% (USDA, 2017). Researchers believe that the population decline of rural America will continue. However, rural communities with environmental resources or close proximity to an urban area may continue to grow in population.

When you hear the term rural America, what do you see? How do you feel? What do you know? For some, rural America is characterized by farming and ranching, small towns, American Indian reservations, or isolated communities. These characteristics are important, yet there are cultural and historical differences in rural America. First, Indigenous peoples of America were the first inhabitants of rural America. Spain, France, England, and Russia colonized America and this resulted in loss of land base, wars, disease, cultural losses, and traumas to Indigenous peoples. Colonization resulted in the Northeast region of rural America being developed in the 1650s. In the mid-1800s, pioneers and miners moved West for the promise of gold, silver, coal, and copper. Rich in minerals, the Western region of the United States continues to provide an excellent source of industry and income for American families. With vastly different histories, the cultures of rural America are unique. These cultures and the history that shaped rural America are critical considerations for rural evaluators.

Evaluation

Most of us have our own definition of **evaluation**. For some, it might be finding the value or worth of something; for others, it might be determining merit or quality, or both value and merit. The history of the term evaluation comes from the French word evaluation, meaning "to find value". This term has been used since 1755 (Online Etymology Dictionary, 2018). In this textbook, we will use the American Evaluation Association's definition of evaluation, "Evaluation is a systematic approach for determining the value of something" (AEA, 2014). There are many uses for evaluation; in this textbook, we will focus on evaluation in rural America. Most evaluation in rural America is program focused—to improve a program, find value, inform policy, and support funding based on short- and long-term results. The term **evaluand** represents what is being evaluated (i.e. a program, service, training, organization, process, or intervention). Often, evaluation is used to address a social problem, a disparity, or a need—because of this use, evaluators are in a unique position to influence social change.

Who is an evaluator? A planner, educator, writer, program facilitator, and problem-solver. Sometimes, evaluators are viewed as judges, educators, or methodologists.

What are their qualifications? Varied, although typically, evaluators have a college degree, social science research skills, strong data analysis skills (qualitative and quantitative), and professional writing abilities.

What do evaluators do? Communicate effectively, maintain professional credibility, practice effective interpersonal skills, know and observe ethical and legal requirements, navigate political issues, design and implement evaluations, analyze and report findings, and follow up and manage evaluations.

Where do they work? At universities; in local and county programs; in private for-profit organizations; for nonprofit organizations, federal agencies, and local extension agencies; and as independent contractors and small business owners.

In the 1980s, the field and practice of evaluation was dominated by psychologists and social science researchers. By the mid-1980s, other disciplines entered the field of evaluation. Guba and Lincoln identified this shift as fourth-generation evaluation (1989), and their book was the impetus for a new generation of evaluation based on the concerns of a community or stakeholder group and the information that is needed to address these concerns.

Rural evaluation

In this textbook, we use the term **rural community evaluation** to refer to evaluation that occurs in a rural context, for rural communities, and with rural populations. Program evaluations are developed for a specific program, with attention to context, goals, resources, and challenges. In rural communities, the evaluation process is unique because of the population, cultures, and location of the community.

Rural evaluators use a variety of methods to evaluate programs, interventions, services, and policies. In this book, we will learn more about several participatory evaluation methods. **Empowerment Evaluation** utilizes 10 principles to empower communities from conceptualization to implementation with a high degree of community ownership and accountability (Fetterman & Wandersman, 2005). **Utilization Focused Evaluation** is focused on the usefulness of an evaluation to the intended users (Patton, 2008). **Real-World Evaluation** provides practical strategies for ensuring the highest-quality evaluation based on context (Bamberger, Rugh, & Mabry, 2011). **Culturally Responsive Evaluation** is a set of strategies used to ensure that culture and context are part of the evaluation (Hood, Hopson, & Kirkhart, 2015).

Indigenous Focused Evaluation was developed by Indigenous peoples, with the goal of focusing on the culture of Indigenous people and their values, history, and postcolonial experience in the United States (LaFrance & Nichols, 2008).

Paradigms

Most of the evaluation methods noted previously are based in a constructivist paradigm. A **paradigm** is a way of looking at the world, a perspective that is value driven (Wall, 2013). A **constructivist paradigm** is based on the belief that each individual creates their own reality, and there are multiple ways to interpret reality; sometimes, the constructivist paradigm is also called interpretivism. A related paradigm that resonates with rural evaluation approaches is a transformative paradigm. **Transformative paradigms**, also called inclusive evaluation, involve community members in the development of the evaluation with the goal of facilitating social change for disadvantaged groups (Mertens, 2014).

Rural communities may have different values and paradigms than evaluators. Can you think of some differences based on what we read earlier? In evaluation (and research), paradigms are important because they influence how activities are carried out and the questions that are asked (Lincoln, Lynham, & Guba, 2011). Yvonna Lincoln, one of the pioneers of new paradigm research, writes, "We are interpretivists, postmodernists, poststructuralists; we are phenomenological, feminist, critical. We choose lenses that are border, racial and ethnic, hybrid, queer, differently abled, indigenous, margin, center" (2010, p. 8).

Examples of programs that have been implemented in rural America include school programs that increase teacher recruitment and retention, employment training programs that increase job skills among the unemployed, single-family housing programs that support affordable housing and home owner-ship in rural America, and rural health-care services outreach programs that increase access to services in rural communities. The paradigm that evaluators use to approach the evaluation and design evaluation question relates to the program goals.

Why a text dedicated to rural evaluation?

To begin, rural communities throughout America are struggling. In the last decade, rural America has experienced population loss. This has led to the reclassification of rural counties due to urbanization (USDA, 2017). Special programs that target the unique needs of rural America often require evaluation. Rural evaluators can play a critical role in revitalizing rural America by documenting community needs, program effectiveness, cost benefit, and policy changes.

Rural evaluators may experience difficulty in measuring outcomes and isolating program impacts from other factors. This text provides information on context, culture, evaluation designs, data collection, analysis, and sustainability that help evaluators determine the outcomes of a rural program.

Finally, there are limited evaluation resources in rural America. This text describes methods of increasing resources and community participation for effective rural evaluation.

The rural evaluation process

Evaluation in rural communities begins with a relationship. This relationship is between the evaluator, the program, and the community. Evaluators play a critical role in helping communities design programs to meet the unique needs of the community. In the rural evaluation process, these four steps can help. We will discuss these steps in greater detail throughout the book:

1. Create a needs assessment that articulates the challenges, strengths, partners, assets, and goals
2. Review evidence for program and determine eligibility
3. Match program to community needs and goals
4. Identify promising models and adapt interventions when necessary.

Evaluators in rural communities often begin the evaluation process early, with the design of a program or service. Evaluators play a crucial role in rural communities; when communities identify a need, evaluators can be there to help them

---

BOX 1.1 Example of a rural solicitation for funding and evaluator's role

Box 1.1—A federal agency posts a funding opportunity in the Federal Register. Rural community programs receive an email notification with a link to the Notice of Solicitation of Applications (NOSA). The Federal Register includes the federal department, branch, title of program, agency, action, summary, and agency contact information. Supplementary information may also be included, with general information and application assistance. The NOSA outlines the minimum and maximum funding amount for each application and the total allocated funds for a given fiscal year. A rural community may contact an evaluator when the NOSA is posted or after a proposal is funded. A rural evaluator works closely with the community to develop the proposal and an evaluation plan for the program. Six months later, the agency sends the community a notice of award (NOA). The NOA is a legal document that is issued to the rural community (grantee). The NOA stipulates the conditions of the grant, reporting requirements, funding amounts, and the budget period. After communities receive a NOA, they begin implementing the funded program. Typically, at this time, evaluators will receive a contract for evaluation services, as outlined in the funded proposal.

Source: Adapted from the Federal Register (2015). Notice of Solicitation of Applications for the Section 533 Housing Preservation Grants for Fiscal Year 2015. Rural Housing Service. Retrieved from https://www.federalregister.gov/documents/2015/05/20/2015-12224/ notice-of-solicitation-of-applications-nosa-for-the-section-533- housing-preservation-grants-for

---

design and evaluate a program to meet that need. Examples of the rural community evaluation process are numerous, as can be seen in Box 1.1.

Implementing, planning, and sustaining rural programs

Implementing programs in rural communities requires a plan. Often, this plan is outlined in the program narrative of a program proposal. Characteristics of successful rural programs include support of local leadership, realistic timelines, adequate funding, political support, and high partner engagement. Challenges are limited resources, isolation, limited access to technology, small populations/ sample sizes, and long distances between rural and urban areas.

Planning evaluation, designing evaluation, identifying measures, and collecting and analyzing data are important steps in rural evaluation. Once a program is designed and implementation is underway, the evaluation begins. Planning evaluation can begin in the development phase of a program or after a project is funded.

Designing the evaluation requires evaluators to engage with stakeholders from a community and then identify which program measures should be monitored in the evaluation. Identifying measures to evaluate requires a close review of funding agency requirements. In the design phase, evaluators identify evaluation questions that they need answered. For example, "What is being evaluated?", "What standards are being used to evaluate a program?", and "How will lessons learned will be used to inform future programs?". Evaluators plan for how data will be collected, analyzed, and reported. We will talk more about evaluating a rural program in Chapter 6.

Sustaining rural programming is difficult, and rural evaluators play a significant role in sustaining rural programs. Begin early in the process; when developing an evaluation plan, identify which efforts should be sustained and how they may be sustained. Begin documenting the resources available, the strategies that have been used in the past to sustain programming, and how these are unique to the rural community. For example, if sustaining a program will require additional grant funding, make sure that the community is eligible, the grant is a good fit for the community, and the community is supportive of continuing the program by seeking additional funds. In this process, it is important to identify resources available and funding opportunities that align with community needs; see rural program resources in this textbook for more information on how to sustain rural programs.

There are various approaches for reaching rural communities with evaluation findings. Documenting the results of a program through rural evaluation is one of the most powerful things that evaluators can do. In essence, the evaluator is the storyteller, the narrator of what took place during a given time and for a specific purpose. Too often, the story gets lost. In this textbook, you will learn the basics of evaluation in rural communities so that you can tell the story in a way that is powerful, transformative, and meaningful.

Summary

Now that we have a basic understanding of terms, evaluation processes, and purpose, we will move to a discussion about context. Context is everything. Being familiar with context helps evaluators plan programs, design evaluations, and interpret results. Evaluations designed acontextually are not valid or reliable. Context matters, and it matters even more in rural community evaluation efforts.

Points to remember

1. There are different definitions for the term "rural". Understanding these definitions is an important first step for evaluators and for determining needs, program eligibility, and resources available.
2. Evaluation has been around for a long time; it has evolved to include multiple disciplines, perspectives, paradigms, and approaches. Selecting the right evaluation approach for rural community valuation requires community engagement and participation.

3. Rural evaluation begins with a relationship between the evaluator and the community. If you do not have a relationship, you cannot be effective as an evaluator.
4. Unique challenges and strengths or rural community evaluation are not unsurmountable, but they do require an understanding that begins with reading this book.

Additional reading and resources

On Evaluation Definitions
American Evaluation Association (ND). *Evaluation Definitions*. Retrieved from http://www.eval.org/p/cm/ld/fid=1

On Rural Classifications
United States Census Bureau (ND). *Metropolitan and Metropolitan Resources*. Retrieved from https://www.census.gov/programs-surveys/metro-micro.html

Defining Rural at the US Census Bureau (2016). *American Community Survey.* https://www.census.gov/content/dam/Census/library/publications/2016/acs/acsgeo-1.pdf

On the History of Rural America
Riney-Kehrberg, P. (Ed.). (2016). *The Routledge History of Rural America.* Routledge.

On the Goldsmith Standard
Goldsmith, Puskin, and Stiles. (2013). *Improving the Operational Definitions of "Rural Areas" for Federal Programs by the Federal Office of Rural Health Policy 2013.* Retrieved from https://www.ruralhealthinfo.org/pdf/improving-the-operational-definition-of-rural-areas.pdf

Chapter questions

1. List the three federal government programs that have unique definitions for the term "rural".
2. Compare and contrast the three separate definitions of rural. How are they similar, and how are they different?
3. What are the four basic steps that can guide the rural evaluation process?
4. List the participatory evaluation methods. Can you think of other participatory evaluation methods that would be appropriate for rural evaluation?

Practice

1. Compare the US Census Bureau definition of rural with those of the Office of Management and Budget, and the Federal Office of Rural Health Policy. How are these definitions similar? How are they different? As a rural evaluator, why is it important to know the different definitions of rural?

2. Identify a rural community in the United States. What is the history of this community? When was this community established? By whom? Has the population declined or increased in the last decade? What are the possible reasons for this change (if any)? How has the history of this community shaped its culture?

3. Consider the term "Evaluation". Write five different sentences using the words "evaluate" or "evaluation".

References

American Evaluation Association (2014). *What is evaluation?* Retrieved from https://www.eval.org/p/bl/et/blogid=2&blogaid=4

Bamberger, M., Rugh, J., & Mabry, L. (2011). *RealWorld evaluation: Working under budget, time, data, and political constraints.* Thousand Oaks, CA: Sage Publications.

Eng, E., & Parker, E. A. (1994). Measuring community competence in the Mississippi Delta: The interface between program evaluation and empowerment. *Health Education Quarterly, 21,* 199–220.

Federal Register (2015). *Notice of Solicitation of Applications for the Section 533 Housing Preservation Grants for Fiscal Year 2015.* Rural Housing Service. Retrieved from https://www.federalregister.gov/documents/2015/05/20/2015-12224/notice-of-solicitation-of-applications-nosa-for-the-section-533-housing-preservation-grants-for

Fetterman, D. M., & Wandersman, A. (2005). *Empowerment evaluation principles in practice.* New York, NY: Guilford Press.

Goldsmith, H., Puskin, D., & Stiles, D. (2013). *Improving the operational definitions of "rural areas" for federal programs by the Federal Office of Rural Health Policy 2013.* Retrieved from https://www.ruralhealthinfo.org/pdf/improving-the-operational-definition-of-rural-areas.pdf

Guba, E. G., & Lincoln, Y. S. (1989). *Fourth generation evaluation.* Newbury Park, CA: Sage Publications.

Health Resources & Services Administration (2017). *Federal Office of Rural Health Policy, Defining the Rural Population.* Retrieved from https://www.hrsa.gov/rural-health/about-us/definition/index.html

Hood, S., Hopson, R. K., & Kirkhart, K. E. (2015). *Culturally responsive evaluation. Theory, practice, and future implications.* In K. A. Newcomer, H. P. Hatry, & J. S. Wholey (Eds.), *In Handbook of Practical Program Evaluation* (4th ed., pp. 281–317). Hoboken NJ: Jossey-Bass

LaFrance, J., & Nichols, R. (2008). Reframing evaluation: Defining an Indigenous evaluation framework. *The Canadian Journal of Program Evaluation, 23*(2), 13.

Lincoln, Y. (2010). "What a long, strange trip it's been": Twenty-five years of qualitative and new paradigm research. *Qualitative Inquiry, 16*(1), 3–9, p. 8.

Lincoln, Y. S., Lynham, S. A., & Guba, E. G. (2011). Paradigmatic controversies, contradictions, and emerging confluences, revisited. In *The Sage handbook of qualitative research* (Vol. 4, pp. 97–128). Thousand Oaks, CA: Sage.

Mertens, D. M. (2014). *Research and evaluation in education and psychology: Integrating diversity with quantitative, qualitative, and mixed methods.* Thousand Oaks, CA: Sage Publications.

Murphy, J. W. (2014). *Community-based interventions: Philosophy and action.* New York, NY: Springer.

Online Etymology Dictionary (2018). *Evaluation (noun).* Retrieved from https://www.etymonline.com/search?q=evaluation

Patton, M. Q. (2008). *Utilization-focused evaluation*. Thousand Oaks, CA: Sage Publications.

Riney-Kehrberg, P. (Ed.). (2016). *The Routledge history of rural America*. New York, NY: Routledge.

United States Census (2017). *One in five Americans live in rural areas*. Retrieved from https://www.census.gov/library/stories/2017/08/rural-america.html

United States Department of Agriculture (2017). Rural America at a Glance 2017 Edition. *Economic Information Bulletin 182*. Retrieved from https://www.ers.usda.gov/webdocs/publications/85740/eib182_brochure%20format.pdf?v=43054

Wall, L. (2013). *Issues in evaluation of complex social change programs for sexual assault prevention (ACSSA Issues No. 14)*. Melbourne: Australian Centre for the Study of Sexual Assault, Australian Institute of Family Studies. Retrieved from https://aifs.gov.au/publications/issues-evaluation-complex-social-change-programs-sexual-assault-preven

2

CONTEXT OF RURAL COMMUNITY EVALUATION

Flying, driving, hiking, and finding—this is one of the best ways that I can describe the context and geography of rural evaluation. Throughout the years, snowstorms, floods, unnamed streets, and free range cows and horses have defined the geography of rural America and left impressions about what and where rural America is.

Context and place

Merriam-Webster defines *context* as the interrelated conditions in which something occurs or exists. This term was first used in the early 15th century meaning "the weaving together of words in language" (ND, para. 2). Context is about circumstances, conditions, surroundings, and environment. The rural evaluation context is different from evaluation in urban areas. Because context is concerned with "place", the first distinguishing characteristic of rural America is the geography. Previous research has established place as a significant demographic factor that directly relates to who lives in rural America. In Chapter 1, we discussed the population and location of rural America. We know that between 72 percent and 84 percent of the land area in the United States is considered rural (Health Resources & Services Administration, 2016), and approximately 15–18 percent of the population live in rural America.

The vast geography of rural America presents unique challenges for rural evaluators. Transportation and travel in and out of rural communities can be difficult. Most rural communities are on a road system, with the exception of some communities in Alaska, but sometimes roads are not enough (Box 2.1).

BOX 2.1 Field notes on context

Early in my evaluation career, I was working in a rural Montana community of about 1,500 people. Located 120 miles away from the nearest major store, this rural community was simply beautiful. On my first visit to the community, there was a major snowstorm. The local weather channel was calling for gusts of 40 miles per hour winds and snow accumulations of 6 inches or more over the following 24 hours. I woke up that morning, knowing that I had to show up in the community—relationships are everything in rural evaluation, and I wanted the community to know that I was dependable, that I could get anywhere at any time, in any circumstance.

I left my home, which was about 140 miles from the rural community. I drove my old truck on backcountry roads, through ice, wind, and white-out conditions, and freezing temperatures. After three hours on the road, I finally arrived. I drove into town and stopped at the only stop light in the entire community. I did not see a car, a person, or even a light on in the buildings. I could not call anyone because I did not have cell reception. So, I parked in front of the program's building and waited. I waited for three hours. The sun came out, ice on the roads began to melt, and our meeting started.

It has been 14 years since I made that trip. I know the community and the context now. I know that in a blizzard, things shut down for a while. People stay inside when the roads are bad and the conditions are unsafe. Rescheduling a meeting or being late to a meeting due to poor driving conditions is part of rural evaluation in the wintertime.

Place also contributes to challenges with communication. In most rural communities, in-person communications are the preferred method of working and establishing relationships between evaluator and community—at times this can be difficult. Consider your travel budget as a rural evaluator, if you do not have a budget and live outside of the community, in another town or state, travel to and from the community can be expensive, and at times difficult.

Characteristics of rural America

What does evaluation really look like in rural communities? How is it different than urban evaluation, and what are some of the similarities? In this chapter, we will discuss the characteristics of rural communities, resources available, social context, political context, employment, poverty, and culture, and how these factors shape the rural evaluation process. Remember, context is everything in rural evaluation. If we don't know context, it is difficult to understand programs, how they work, and how to evaluate them.

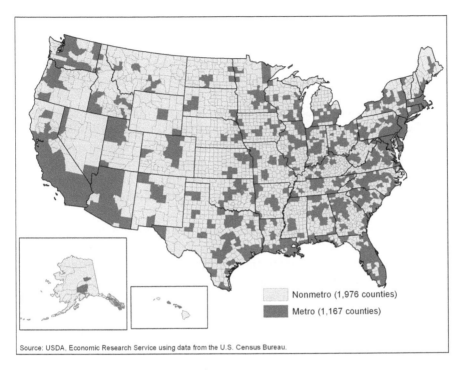

FIGURE 2.1   Image USDA Metro and Nonmetro.

Who lives in rural America?

Community characteristics/population density. We learned in Chapter 1 that the term rural refers to communities with less than 2,500 residents. Sometimes the terms metro and nonmetro are used to define rural areas in America. The United States Department of Agriculture (USDA) map of metro and nonmetro counties from 2013 shows that most nonmetro counties are located in the Midwest, North Central, and Western parts of the United States (Figure 2.1).

Rural America: three types of communities

Researchers Ulrich-Schad and Duncan identified three types of rural American communities: amenity rich, transitioning, and chronically poor (2018). Amenity-rich rural American communities are increasing in population size, and they often have natural amenities, like lakes, mountains, and oceans that attract residents who want an outdoor lifestyle. Transitioning rural areas are highly dependent on agriculture, timber, and manufacturing. Population growth and decline in transitioning rural areas is mixed. The third type of rural America is the chronically poor. These are areas located in counties throughout Appalachia and the rural south. These areas have experienced population loss over a long period of time and struggle with poverty, isolation, and limited education (Ulrich-Schad & Duncan, 2018).

Depopulation, deaths, diversity

We also know that the population of rural America is changing. This presents challenges for rural America and programming efforts. Daniel Lichter is a Cornell University researcher and describes these changes as the three "D's" of rural population change: they are depopulation, deaths, and diversity (Lichter, 2017). **Depopulation** refers to the rural population decline that is occurring right now. **Deaths** are due to natural decreases where there are more deaths in rural America than births. **Diversity** refers to the increase in racial minorities and immigrants in rural America, namely Native American, African American, and Hispanic (Lichter, 2017). The aging and diverse populations of rural America also present unique medical, legal, and social service needs that are important for rural evaluators and programs to recognize.

Since 2010, most rural communities have experienced a population loss (Thiede, Brown, Sanders, Glasgow, & Kulscar, 2017). The declining population of rural America directly relates to the number of economic opportunities in a given community. In urban areas, there is a large enough population to support basic amenities and services, but in rural areas, there is a lack of basic services to sustain a population. The lack of amenities and basic services in some rural American communities has resulted in a chronic outmigration of the population.

Rural populations

Rural populations are more likely to be older and male than urban populations (Fuguitt, Brown, & Beale, 1989). They are also more likely to be married, and live in their birth state than urban populations. Rural adults are less likely to have a college education. The poverty rate of rural adults is slightly less than that of urban adults (11.7 percent vs. 14.0 percent), and rural adults are slightly more likely to have insurance than urban adults. Children in rural America are slightly more likely to be uninsured than urban children (7.3 percent vs. 6.3 percent). More people in rural America own homes compared to those in urban America, although internet access in rural America is still lagging behind urban areas. Twenty-three percent of households do not have access to the internet (US Census Bureau, 2016) (Table 2.1).

Other unique population characteristics in rural America include a disproportionate number of veterans living in rural communities. Twenty-four percent of all veterans currently live in rural America compared with 18% of the total population (Kleykamp, 2017).

Health

Health disparities are significant among rural Americans. Rates of preventable diseases, like obesity, diabetes, cancer, and injury, are higher in rural America (Eberhardt & Pamuk, 2004). Rural American populations also experience health disparities related to high-risk health behaviors including smoking, limited physical activity, poor diet, and limited use of seatbelts. Fewer rural Americans are covered by Medicare for drug coverage, and rural Americans have less access to physicians and specialists. Rural adults are more likely to describe their health as fair or poor than urban adults. However, the life expectancy for males and females living in rural America is higher than urban areas (Table 2.2) (National Rural Health Association, 2018a).

TABLE 2.1 Differences between Rural and Urban Populations

	Rural	*Urban*
Adults (18+ years)		
Median age	51 years	45 years
Now married	61.9%	50.8%
Lives in birth state	65.4%	48.3%
Bachelor's degree or higher	19.5%	29.0%
Civilian employed	67.6%	70.0%
Poverty rate	11.7%	14.0%
Uninsured rate	13.6%	15.3%
Children		
Percent of total population	22.3%	23.5%
Poverty rate	18.9%	22.3%
Uninsured rate	7.3%	6.3%
Housing and households		
Median income	$52,386	$54,296
Home ownership rate	81.1%	59.8%
No internet access	23.8%	17.3%

Source: US Census Bureau (2016).

TABLE 2.2 National Rural and Urban Health Comparison

	Rural	*Urban*
Percentage of population	19.3%	80.7%
Number of physicians per 10,000 people	13.1	31.2
Number of specialists per 100,000 people	30	263
Population aged 65 and older	18%	12%
Adults who describe health status as fair/poor	19.5%	15.6%
Adolescents who smoke	11%	5%
Male life expectancy in years	76.2	74.1
Female life expectancy	81.3	79.7
Percentage of dual-eligible Medicare beneficiaries	30%	70%
Medicare beneficiaries without drug coverage	43%	27%
Percentage covered by Medicaid	16%	13%

Source: National Rural Health Association (2018).

The National Rural Health Association discussed rural health in their 2018 article:

> The obstacles faced by health care providers and patients in rural areas are vastly different than those in urban areas. Economic factors, cultural and social differences, educational shortcomings, lack of recognition by legislators and the sheer isolation of living in remote areas all conspire to create health care disparities and impede rural Americans in their struggle to lead normal, healthy lives.
>
> *(National Rural Health Association, 2018a, p. 1)*

Rural America has also experienced a larger number of deaths due to the opioid epidemic, suicide, and alcoholism (James, 2017) than more urban areas. Rural populations most affected by higher opioid mortality rates include rural white men and women in their middle ages, rural black Americans, individuals with less than a high school diploma, those who are unemployed, and individuals who experience social and economic disadvantage (James, 2017).

Employment and economy

What employment and economic opportunities are available in rural America?

Rural America is unique in that employment and economic opportunities are largely linked to agriculture, mining, and manufacturing (Carr & Kefalas, 2009). However, in the last decade, employment and economic opportunities have declined in most of rural America. This has contributed to a population loss, especially of younger people who move to more urban areas to find jobs, attend school, and access resources not available in rural America (Cowan, 2001). High rates of unemployment and population loss challenge employment and economic opportunities. Many rural residents move to urban areas to seek employment and higher wages.

Agriculture, lower wage jobs, limited year-round work, and less education are characteristics of rural employment and economy in rural America. Rural communities have not fully recovered from the Great Recession that started in December 2007 and ended for most communities, in June 2009. Rural communities remain below their prerecession employment levels and a report by the Bureau of Labour and Statistics indicates that there are 770,000 fewer jobs in October 2017 than in October 2007 (Henderson, 2017). In comparison, job growth in urban areas has improved, with nine million more jobs in 2017 than in 2007, but 88% of these jobs are in urban areas (Henderson, 2017). The effects of the recession in rural communities are still evident today. The declining and flat population growth results in lower purchasing power, fewer consumers, and fewer organizations available to build programs. The limited growth results in lower tax base and reduces public funds available for programming. More rural communities are seeking additional funding through state, federal, local, and nonprofit agencies to support community-based programs. These grants and programs often require evaluation and evaluators with a knowledge of rural context and community.

Poverty

What do we know about poverty in rural America?

Poverty rates vary by region and rural locations. Rural America experiences more poverty than urban America. Rural poverty in the southern region of the United States is 21.3% compared with 15.5% of the urban population in the southern region (ERS, 2018). Factors that contribute to rural poverty include deindustrialization in the 1980s and an increase in the number of Hispanic people living in the United States in the 1990s and 2000s. Hispanic populations experience poverty at a higher rate than non-Hispanic Whites (ERS, 2018). Poverty contributes to food insecurity, substance abuse, and limited access to health. Poverty is 10% higher among female-headed households in rural areas than it is in urban areas.

Child poverty

According to the Economic Research Service, 23.5% of rural children in the United States were poor in 2016 (ERS, 2018). In comparison, 20.5% of urban children in the United States were poor (ERS, 2018). Child poverty rates vary by county, although of the 41 counties in the United States with child poverty rates greater than 50%, 38 were in rural counties. Counties with the highest child poverty rates were Mellette County, SD, 70.9%; Issaquena County, MS, at 68.7%; and East Carroll Parish, LA, at 68.4%. Child poverty rates in some areas of the United States are persistently higher among African American children (ERS, 2018).

Persistent poverty

Persistent poverty is used to define counties who have experienced poverty for more than 30 years. The US federal law definition of poverty from 2011 is "20 percent or more of its population has lived in poverty over the past 30 years" (Dalaker, 2017). During the Obama administration, 301 rural counties were identified as suffering from persistent poverty compared with just 51 non-rural counties (Martin, 2016).

Technology, health care, education, and natural resources

Technology, health-care, education, and natural resources are what make rural American unique. Understanding the availability of these resources in rural America is an important step in planning and implementing rural evaluation.

Technology

Rural America experiences limited access to technology and digital knowledge-based systems. Modern high-speed telecommunications, computer systems and internet for personal and business needs are often not available. An estimated 24% of rural Americans do not have internet access in their homes, compared with 17% of urban American households (US Census Bureau, 2016). Limited access to technology presents unique challenges for evaluators. In communities with access to the internet, evaluators can leverage this as a resource to increase the reach of resources available to a community—provide online trainings, webinars, and programming support.

Health care

Health care in rural America is a major problem. Rural populations have less access to health care than urban populations. Rural populations may not have the funds to pay for services or have insurance coverage. Some may not have transportation to and from the clinic. Others may not speak English and experience difficulty in voicing their health concerns with a provider (Rural Health Information Hub, 2017). Efforts to address health care in rural American are underway, yet the problems remain—people living in rural America experience health disparities related to place, that could be alleviated through policy reform that ensures health care and health access for all. Effective rural evaluation can inform policy and increase health-care access.

Education

Despite lower educational attainment of rural Americans, the education systems located throughout rural America are a tremendous resource. Rural schools account for more than half of America's educational system (Martin, 2016). Yet, rural schools must advocate for funding to address the lingering effects of generational poverty, food scarcity, and limited job and employment opportunities. Rural schools play an important role in shaping local economies, changing policy, and promoting equity. However, a major challenge facing rural communities is that rural students are less likely to attend college than urban students. One of the main reasons that rural students do not go on to college is the cost.

Natural resources

Compared with other countries, the United States encompasses a large land mass. Rich in natural resources, the United States has quality farmland, lakes, rivers, streams, oil, coal, and gas. Many of these natural resources are located throughout rural America. These resources impact how communities interact, when they interact, and the kinds of social activities that are available in a community.

Social context of rural America

Chances are you have been to rural America. You might have noticed the social context. When we use the terms social context, this means the physical and social setting of rural America—where people live, communicate, learn, and socialize. The social context also includes culture.

Rural America social context is different than urban areas because of the limited number of resources and the smaller population. Here are some differences that may be useful as you begin thinking about social context in rural America.

- Churches may be the only institution in a rural community.
- Local libraries often fill a niche for programming by providing access to outlying rural communities.
- Grocery stores, community boards, gas stations, and Lions and Elks Club serve as communication hubs.
- Basketball games, dances, and other school-based events are social events, in rural communities these events are places to connect with friends and get caught up on current events. Unlike urban America where hundreds or thousands of people may attend, rural America schools and events are attended by individuals in a community who often know one another.
- Although isolated and often distant, rural communities are close-knit with a strong sense of identity and kinship systems.
- Rural community members may be more willing to help others in times of need.

The social context includes the culture of rural America. **Culture** refers to the values, and shared characteristics of a particular group. Sociologist Ann Swidler views culture as a tool kit of symbols, stories, rituals, and worldviews that we collect over our lifetime based on our experiences (1986).

Defining the culture of rural America requires an understanding of the people who make up rural America and what they value. In a 2017 survey by the Washington Post-Kaiser Family Foundation, most adults living in rural America indicated they feel that their values are different than people who live in big cities (DelReal & Clement, 2017). In some rural communities, this translates to more conservative views of religion, politics, and economics.

Political context in rural America

Evaluation is by nature, political. Navigating the political landscape of rural America requires an understanding of what the political climate is and the role of evaluators in politics. There are four main aspects of politics in rural America that evaluators must recognize.

First, evaluations may involve politically charged topics and people who are passionate about the issue, and evaluators must align themselves with the views of the community and, to the extent possible, support the community's views and stance on a given political issue. Evaluation efforts must show value, and values influence political views—these can result in conflicts about what is most important or how to achieve a program goal or task. Donna Mertens (2015) writes, "The direct relationship between evaluation of social and educational programs and access to resources sets the stage for tensions that can sometimes result in conflicts" (p. 47).

Second, evaluators must understand the political divide between urban and rural communities and how this impacts evaluation efforts. There has always been a political divide between rural and urban Americans, but in the present day it seems to growing. The most recent presidential election in the United States was won by the white rural American vote, more than 62% of rural and small town America voted for Trump (Morin, 2016). According to a survey by the Pew Research Center in June 2016, rural whites were more concerned about job opportunities, immigrants working in the United States, and a lower standard of living for their children. The Pew Research Center survey also found differences in how rural and urban voters view education and the role of higher education. Morin (2016) writes:

> rural white men stand apart from rural women as well as from white urban and suburban residents. While substantial majorities of men and women see some role for colleges and universities in providing necessary skills and education, rural white men are far less likely than rural white women (71% vs. 92%) to say this. Rural white men are also significantly less likely than urban or suburban white men (82% and 84%, respectively) to see a role for institutions of higher education.

Katherine Cramer, author of the *Politics of Resentment*, further describes the rural–urban political divide and the growing economic inequality that contributes to differences in power, influence, and quality of life (2016). Cramer reports three feelings that rural communities have in common: (1) decision makers and policy makers ignore rural areas, (2) rural areas receive fewer resources than urban areas, and (3) rural communities have values and a way of life that is misunderstood by urban people (2016). Cramer coined the term rural consciousness, meaning to identify with rural people and rural places.

Third, evaluators must recognize the different leadership and governance structure in place that support local rural programs and services. Rural communities may have special districts for schools, fire protection, sanitary services, public transportation, public libraries, and natural resource management. State and local leaders are a foundation of rural America and advocate for policy and funding to support rural districts and needs. US Senator Cory Gardner represented northeastern Colorado as a lawmaker and congressman (Frank, 2017). In a December 2017 interview with the Denver Post, Cory Gardner shared this perspective:

If you're a rural policymaker, you have to understand what's happening in the urban areas because they drive so much of the business and the conversation of the state. But, if you're an urban legislator or urban policymaker, you don't have to pay attention to what's happening in those rural areas.

In addition to state political leaders, local governments like city councils often lead programming and development efforts in rural communities. Local governments in rural communities follow state rather than federal law in most cases. They include county governments, town or townships governments, municipal governments, and special purpose governments. However, some rural areas do not have a municipal government below the county level. In some instances, cities and counties work together as a single municipal government. Some states have regional Councils of Government (North Carolina) that serve regional areas and serve as a unified voice for the people.

Fourth, American Indian and Alaska Native political contexts are unique because they are sovereign nations (Biolsi, 2005). Chief Justice Marshall of the United States Supreme Court shared this perspective, "Indian Nations had always been considered as distinct, independent political communities, retaining their original natural rights, as the undisputed possessors of the soil…The very term 'nation' so generally applied to them means 'a people distinct from others'" (NCAI, p. 6).

There are 567 federally recognized tribal entities in the contiguous 48 states and Alaska (Indian Affairs Bureau, 2017). Nearly half (239) of these federally recognized tribes are located in Alaska, while the remaining 328 are located in 35 other states (NCAI, 2018). Tribes are governed by elected or appointed leaders who serve constituents as advocates, policy makers, reformers, and visionaries for social change. Tribal governments are responsible for basic infrastructure like roads, emergency services, and law enforcement. Tribal governments also work to build local reservation economics while advocating for education and self-sufficiency. The Native American Caucus of the California Democratic Party writes:

> Tribal governments are the oldest governments in existence in the Western Hemisphere. Despite common misperceptions, the United States was not the first government to institute democratic rule and introduce concepts of fair representation, equality, and justice for all. At a time when European governments were authoritarian and hierarchical, traditional tribal governments were based upon principles of democracy, equality, freedom, and respect.
>
> *(p. 1)*

Conducting evaluations with American Indian or Alaska Native tribes requires a different set of approvals and political involvement. Evaluators may interact with elected tribal leaders, and in most cases get their approval before beginning work in the community or with a tribal program. Findings from evaluations may be directed to tribal leaders, because they have the power to influence change, improve policy, and advocate for additional funding. Evaluators must keep in mind that the political context of each tribe is unique. This uniqueness dates back thousands of years based on history, culture, language, tradition, and worldview. Evaluators must seek out opportunities to understand the political structure while honoring the protocols for doing evaluation in American Indian and Alaska Native communities.

In summary, navigating the political context in rural America requires an understanding of the community, context, culture, and needs (see more in Chapter 3: Culturally Competent Research and Evaluation). Rural evaluators benefit from working with local leaders, community advocates, and local governments.

Rural context-focused evaluation

Rural context requires a rural-focused evaluation. Rural populations may not trust outsiders coming into a community to do evaluation. Understanding the context of rural America will help evaluators build trust and develop relationships necessary for effective evaluation. There is limited funding and resources available for rural communities. This means that we need to develop programming and interventions that are most effective and efficient—rural evaluators can help achieve this. The sociopolitical context of rural America is unique and could benefit from a rural-focused evaluation. Finally, the knowledge that exists in the community may be different than published evidence from urban settings.

A significant argument for rural-focused evaluation relates to the results and recommendations from a given program. When a rural-focused evaluation is used, the results are more relevant, valid, reliable, and replicable (Box 2.2).

BOX 2.2 A call for rural-focused evaluation

Consider an evaluation that is developed by an external evaluator at a major university in an urban area. The evaluator may be interested in publishing, testing a method or a theory, or building a research base about a rural community. Without substantive input from community, it is likely that results of the evaluation will not be relevant, valid, or reliable. This text advocates for a rural-focused evaluation approach based on rural community needs and rural community resources and strengths. Focusing on these areas will ensure maximum benefit to the community and translation of results into meaningful outcomes.

Summary

In this chapter, we have covered a lot of ground, we are building on the context of rural America because this understanding will help you as a rural evaluator. We learned that place is a primary factor in rural evaluation context and is connected to every characteristic found in a rural community. In this chapter, we also discussed the importance of factors like social and political context, poverty, culture, resources available, and the economic landscape of rural America. As we end this chapter on context, I encourage you to reflect on your knowledge and experiences in rural America. How has context shaped the work that you are doing, how you communicate with others, where you meet, and what you do?

Points to remember

1. Context matters in rural evaluation.
2. Rural populations experience disparities in health education, and access to health care.
3. Rural America social context is different than urban areas because there are fewer resources and a smaller population.
4. The urban–rural political divide is growing; most adults living in rural America feel that their values are different than people who live in big cities. In some rural communities, this translates to more conservative views of religion, politics, and economics. Evaluators must be thoughtful in how they approach these views and differences.
5. The political structure of rural America is unique, ranging from local governments to elected tribal councils and sovereignty. Evaluators must know the political structure and honor it.

Additional reading and resources

On USDA Frontier and Remote Area Codes
United States Department of Agriculture Economic Research Service (2016). Frontier and Remote Area Codes. Retrieved from www.ers.usda.gov/data-products/frontier-and-remote-area-codes/

On Education
National Center for Education Statistics. (ND). Rural Education in America. Retrieved from https://nces.ed.gov/surveys/ruraled/

On Health Disparities
Bennett, K, Bankole, Olatosi, & Probst, J (2008). Health Disparities: A Rural-Urban Chartbook by the South Carolina Rural Health Research Center.

On Leadership, Research, and Politics

Pew Research Center (ND). US Politics and Policy. Retrieved from http://www.people-press.org/

Center for Rural Affairs (ND). Leadership for Rural Communities. http://www.cfra.org/resources/leaders

Chapter questions

1. Compare and contrast the urban and rural population of the United States.
2. List the differences in health-care access in rural vs. urban communities.
3. Review Table 2.1, and summarize the primary health differences in rural compared with urban populations. Are any of these differences surprising? What might contribute to these differences?
4. What is meant by the term Rural Divide? As a rural evaluator, why is it important to understand the rural divide?
5. Describe the political landscape of rural America. How might this challenge you as an evaluator? What if your political views are different from the population that you are working in and with?

Practice

1. Go to the United States Department of Agriculture Economic Research Service website (www.ers.usda.gov/data-products/atlas-of-rural-and-small-town-america/go-to-the-atlas.aspx). Review the map by selecting Map to Display. Note the different categories that you can select, people, jobs, county classifications, income, and veterans. You can also search by keyword. Select county classifications and the rural–urban continuum code. Review the number of counties that are completely rural. Review the number of counties that are metro with a population of one million or more. Zoom into the state and county that you live in. Explore other variables from the drop-down list to learn more about community poverty, population change, and jobs. How might you use these data as a rural evaluator? What are some limitations to the data?
2. Go to the Rural Health Information Hub website (https://www.rural-healthinfo.org/topics/healthcare-access). Review information on rural health access. Why is access to health care important for rural Americans? What are some of the efforts in place to improve health-care access in rural America? Describe health-care services that are most difficult to access in rural communities due to lack of quality or limited providers. How might a rural evaluator work with a community to address these problems?
3. Learn more about tribal sovereignty and governance. The National Congress of American Indians was established in 1944 to serve the broad interests of tribal governments and communities (http://www.ncai.org/). Review current initiatives, news, and events.

References

Biolsi, T. (2005). Imagined geographies: Sovereignty, indigenous space, and American Indian struggle. *American Ethnologist, 32*(2), 239–259.

Carr, P. J., & Kefalas, M. J. (2009). *Hollowing out the middle: The rural brain drain and what it means for America.* Boston, MA: Beacon Press.

Cowan, T. (2001). *Changing structure of agriculture and rural America: Emerging opportunities and challenges.* CRS Report for Congress, RL31172, Retrieved from https://www.nationalaglawcenter.org/assests/crs/RL31172.pdf

Cramer, K. (2016). *The politics of resentment. Rural consciousness in Wisconsin and the rise of Scott Walker.* Chicago, IL: Chicago Studies in American Politics.

Dalaker, J. (2017). *The 10–20–30 Rule and persistent poverty counties.* Congressional Research Service. Retrieved from *https://fas.org/sgp/crs/misc/R44748.pdf*

DelReal, J., & Clement, S. (2017). *The rural divide. Washing Post democracy dies in darkness.* Retrieved from https://www.washingtonpost.com/graphics/2017/national/rural-america/?utm_term=.8ae6c2558cb6

Eberhardt, M. S., & Pamuk, E. R. (2004). The importance of place of residence: Examining health in rural and non-rural areas. *American Journal of Public Health, 94*(10), 1682–1686.

Economic Research Service (2018). *Rural poverty and well-being.* United States Department of Agriculture. Retrieved from https://www.ers.usda.gov/topics/rural-economy-population/rural-poverty-well-being.aspx

Frank, J. (2017). *Colorado's growing political divide leaves rural communities feeling forgotten and voiceless. The Denver Post. Interview with Cory Gardner.* Retrieved from https://www.denverpost.com/2017/12/24/colorado-politics-divide-rural-urban-communities-donald-trump/

Fuguitt, G. V., Brown, D. L., & Beale, C. L. (1989). *Rural and small town America.* New York, NY: Russell Sage Foundation.

Health Resources Services Administration (2016). *Federal Office of Rural Health Policy, Defining the rural population.* Retrieved from https://www.hrsa.gov/rural-health/about-us/definition/index.html

Henderson, G. (2017). The recession lingers in rural America. *Ag Web Farm Journal.* Retrieved from https://www.agweb.com/article/recession-lingers-in-rural-america/

Indian Affairs Bureau (2017). *Indian entities recognized and eligible to receive services from the United States Bureau of Indian Affairs.* Federal Register. 82 FR 4915. Retrieved from https://www.federalregister.gov/documents/2017/01/17/2017-00912/indian-entities-recognized-and-eligible-to-receive-services-from-the-united-states-bureau-of-indian

James, W. (2017). *The shifting demographics of rural America: Health and Mortality. Congressional Briefing.* Population Reference Bureau. Retrieved from https://www.prb.org/wp-content/uploads/2017/04/Congressional20Briefing20James20Presentation.pdf

Kleykamp, M. (2017). *The changing demographics of rural America: Veterans.* Congressional Briefing Population Reference Bureau. Retrieved from https://www.prb.org/wp-content/uploads/2017/04/Kleykamp20UMD_PAA20rural20veterans20Powerpoint.pdf

Lichter, D. (2017). *The changing demographics of rural America.* Congressional Briefing Population Reference Bureau. Retrieved from http://www.prb.org/wp-content/uploads/2017/04/Lichter_Rural20Population20Change.pdf

Martin, R. (2016). Salvaging education in rural America. *The Atlantic,* January 5, 2016 Education. Retrieved from https://www.theatlantic.com/education/archive/2016/01/americas-rural-schools/422586/

Merriam-Webster (ND). *Definition and history of context*. Retrieved from https://www.merriam-webster.com/dictionary/context

Mertens, D. M. (2014). *Research and evaluation in education and psychology: Integrating diversity with quantitative, qualitative, and mixed methods*. Thousand Oaks, CA: Sage publications.

Morin, R. (2016). *Behind Trump's win in rural white America: Women joined men in backing him*. Fact Tank News in the Numbers. Pew Research Center. November 17, 2016. Retrieved from http://www.pewresearch.org/fact-tank/2016/11/17/behind-trumps-win-in-rural-white-america-women-joined-men-in-backing-him/

National Congress of American Indians (2018). *Policy issues. Tribal governance*. Chief Justice Marshall US Supreme Court p. 6. Retrieved from https://www.ncai.org/policy-issues/tribal-governance

National Rural Health Association (2018a). *About rural health care*. Retrieved from https://www.ruralhealthweb.org/about-nrha/about-rural-health-care, paragraph 1.

National Rural Health Association (2018b). *Health resources and services administration and rural health information hub*. Retrieved from https://www.ruralhealthweb.org/about-nrha/about-rural-health-care

Native American Caucus of the California Democratic Party (ND). *Tribal Sovereignty: History and the Law*, p. 1. Retrieved from https://www.nativeamericancaucus.org/content/tribal-sovereignty-history-and-law

Rural Health Information Hub (2017). *Healthcare access in rural communities*. Retrieved from https://www.ruralhealthinfo.org/topics/healthcare-access

Swidler, A. (1986). Culture in action: Symbols and strategies. *American Sociological Review*, *51*, 273–286.

Thiede, B. C., Brown, D. L., Sanders, S. R., Glasgow, N., & Kulcsar, L. J. (2017). A demographic deficit? Local population aging and access to services in rural America, 1990–2010. *Rural Sociology*, *82*, 44–74. doi:10.1111/ruso.12117

Ulrich-Schad, J., & Duncan, C. (2018). People and places left behind: Work, culture and politics in the rural United States. *The Journal of Peasant Studies*, *45*(1), 59–79. doi:10.1080/03066150.2017.1410702

US Census Bureau (2016). *2011–2015 American Community Survey, 5-year estimates and 2015 American Community Survey 1-year estimates*. Revised December 8, 2016. Retrieved from https://www.census.gov/library/visualizations/2016/comm/acs-rural-urban.html

3

CULTURAL COMPETENCE IN EVALUATION

I have come to understand what culture is by being in places and with people who have a culture that is different than my own. I have come to know that being culturally responsive in evaluation means more than just identifying a group, a language, a value or a place. It is more than just following standards or checking a box that shows I agree to be culturally competent. Cultural competence in evaluation is about respect, empowerment, transformation, social justice, equity, and meaning.

What is culture?

Evaluators often work in cultures that are not their own. Culture encompasses diversity in views, values, histories, and context. In Chapter 2, we learned that culture is part of the social context of rural America. **Culture** includes **group factors** like social structures and relations, the local economy, resources available, the location and geography, leadership, and policy (Campbell & Jolly, ND). Culture also encompasses **individual factors** including race, ethnicity, religion, language, sexual orientation, age, and gender of rural America (AEA, 2011). You may recall from Chapter 1 that **community** relates to a geographic place or a group with shared values or characteristics. Rural evaluators must embrace culture and understand how it is used throughout the evaluation process. Campbell and Jolly name three things that evaluators need to do when acknowledging the cultural context in evaluation: (1) know and understand the contextual factors that are relevant to the evaluation; (2) know our own worldview and assumptions; and (3) build relationships with the community, and spend time with program staff and participants (ND).

Culture plays an important role in evaluation, especially since evaluation is about finding value, and values are inherently linked to culture. Many rural programs are funded to address a social problem, or a need in the community (Mertens, 2015). Dominant culture can be overpowering and seek to find deficits or needs rather than strengths in rural evaluation. Evaluators must be attentive to culture, and keep the values of a community at the forefront of any evaluation process.

Understanding the terms

Have you noticed that there are different ways in which culture and cultural competence are discussed in evaluation? Part of being a culturally competent evaluator is knowing the language and terms, how they are used and in what context. **Context** is the interrelated condition in which something occurs or exists. This term was first used in the early 15th century meaning, "the weaving together of words in language" (Merriam-Webster, ND, para. 1). **Cultural competence** in evaluation is "a systematic, responsive inquiry that is actively cognizant, understanding, and appreciative of the cultural context in which the evaluation takes place" (SenGupta, Hopson, & Thompson-Robinson, 2004, p. 1). In contrast, cultural responsiveness is a process that explores the value of something (treatment, program, or intervention) based on what is most important to the community that is both culturally and contextually defensible (Kirkhart & Hopson, 2012). **Cross-cultural** refers to the interactions between two or more cultures (Merryfield, 1985) including the evaluator's own culture and that of the community being evaluated. This text uses these culture terms broadly.

Acculturation is a term used to describe individuals who maintain parts of their original culture and accept new cultural norms. Acculturation is impacted by time and migration in rural America, socioeconomic status, connections to culture, and predominant culture within a community.

Multiculturalism involves different cultures or cultural identities within a rural community, state, or nation. Rural communities are often multicultural with different cultures, histories, values, and languages represented. A culturally competent evaluator is aware of these cultures and engages them based on the program requirements and target population.

Linguistic Competence is the capacity of an organization and its personnel to communicate effectively (NCCC, 2018). Linguistic competence in rural communities requires evaluators to communicate in a way that is easy for community members to understand, especially those who may not speak English or individuals who have low literacy skills or a hearing or visual impairment that interferes with their ability to communicate.

Validity in evaluation requires a culturally competent evaluator. Understanding the culture of a community or rural population can help ensure that the evaluation results are valid. The American Evaluation Association reports that validity and cultural competence are supported when evaluations support the life experiences of the program participants or target population, when relationships support communication and trust, when the theory and design of the evaluation rely on culture to interpret findings, when the design and measures used reflect the cultural context, and when the social consequences of an evaluation are considered (AEA, 2011).

Language deals with how we convey information to the world. Bias and stereotypes are often perpetuated through language, reports, and communications. Culturally competent evaluators challenge stereotypes, are accurate in their appraisals and work, and ensure that the evaluation uses the primary or preferred language, communication style, and methods (AEA, 2011).

Power must be acknowledged in evaluation. Pettifor acknowledges that the shift in power benefits disadvantaged groups:

> In the helping professions, the traditional power differential or hierarchy between the expert professional and the compliant recipient is being eroded with concepts of collaboration, normalization, autonomy, and empowerment. For disadvantaged populations there is beginning to be more opportunity to be heard, respected, and to gain more control of their own lives.
>
> *(1999, p. 141)*

The implications of this statement for rural communities are that rural evaluators must seek to balance power, to focus on dismantling the historical hierarchy, and using evaluation as a tool for social change. Culturally competent evaluation addresses power dynamics while ensuring that groups are not marginalized (AEA, 2011). Similarly, rural evaluators must ensure that there is equal power sharing among groups, and that degrees, titles, and status are not used to overpower the evaluation direction or outcomes. Evaluators can promote equality and self-determination through culturally competent evaluation practice (Mertens, 2015).

Why does cultural competence matter in rural communities?

Cultural competence in rural evaluation is necessary because of the unique cultures of rural America. In Chapters 1 and 2, we discussed the rural context and population. We learned that social context includes culture and that culture is defined as the shared values and characteristics of a given group. Values in rural America may differ. For example, Harris, McFarland, Siebold, Aguilar, and Sarmiento (2007) implemented a school-based prevention program in rural Idaho, and report "Adults in each community have a diverse range of attitudes and beliefs about alcohol or other drug use and incidents of violence among young people" (p. 88). Since evaluation seeks to find value, we must first understand the values of a community, culture, or specific group of people.

Can you imagine an evaluation that does not include the culture of the community and population involved in program or service being evaluated? Cultural

---

BOX 3.1 Field notes on culture and adapting instruments

As a rural evaluator working in a reservation community, I was given a published scale to use. This was validated for American Indian populations and was highly recommended by the funding agency that we were working with at the time. I reviewed the scale and the response options. I noticed that some of the statements did not reflect the specific culture of the community that I was working with. For example, one of the questions asked about participation in a cultural ceremony gave the example of a ceremony that was not practiced in that tribe/community. This scale had to be revised by the community and cultural leaders to reflect the kinds of ceremonies that were appropriate for the tribe, the age of respondents, and the language. We can have the best instruments, but if they do not reflect the unique culture of a population, they will not produce valid or reliable results. This is one of just many instances where culturally competent evaluation is important.

---

competence shows in how evaluation plans evolve; how evaluation instruments are developed and adapted; how data are collected and analyzed; and how results are shared with the community, leaders, and funding agencies. Culturally competent evaluators engage stakeholders early in the evaluation planning process. When instruments are developed, evaluators ensure that they are valid for the community in both language, communication styles, norms, and context (Chouinard & Cousins, 2009) (Box 3.1).

Seek involvement

Seek support and involvement from individuals who are part of the culture or familiar with it. Campbell and Jolly acknowledge the importance of culture in their article "Beyond Rigor: In a sea of context":

> An evaluation team needs to include people who are familiar with the major culture groups that have relevance for an evaluation. These may be people who are members of those groups or people who have experience working with those groups. No one can know everything about a culture, much less multiple cultures, but all evaluation team members should have some background knowledge of the relevant culture groups. Knowing such basics as appropriate levels of formality in language and dress, how people are addressed, and what behaviors are considered rude can make a big difference on the evaluation—especially the data collection.
>
> (ND, p. 4)

Guiding principles for rural evaluators

The American Evaluation Association Cultural Competence in Evaluation Task Force recognizes the importance of cultural competence in evaluation and in their 2011 position statement wrote:

> To ensure recognition, accurate interpretation, and respect for diversity, evaluators should ensure that the members of the evaluation team collectively demonstrate cultural competence. Cultural competence is a stance taken toward culture, not a discrete status or simple mastery of particular knowledge and skills. A culturally competent evaluator is prepared to engage with diverse segments of communities to include cultural and contextual dimensions important to the evaluation. Culturally competent evaluators respect the cultures represented in the evaluation throughout the process.
>
> *(2011, para. 4)*

Then, in 2013, the American Evaluation Association convened a task force to explore the ethics in evaluation that would support culturally competent evaluation. These ethics are guiding principles based on Western cultures in the United States. Rural evaluators may need to modify these principles to fit differences in "culture, religion, gender, disability, age, sexual orientation, and ethnicity" (AEA, 2013, p. 22). Let's review American Evaluation Association's (AEA) five principles in more detail.

1. Systematic Inquiry: Evaluators conduct systematic, data-based inquiries.

In rural evaluation, this means that the evaluation approach is based on the highest standards available for the population. Communicating results should be done in contextually appropriate manner.

2. Competence: Evaluators provide competent performance to stakeholders.

In rural evaluation it is important that evaluators have the appropriate experience and education to carry out an evaluation. Evaluators must be culturally competent, understanding that their own worldviews may be different than the rural community or target population. Evidence of cultural competence may be in the diversity of *race, ethnicity, gender, religion, language, history, or socioeconomic status*.

3. Integrity/Honesty: Evaluators display honesty and integrity in their own behavior, and attempt to ensure the honesty and integrity of the entire evaluation process.

Rural evaluators must ensure that they have no conflict of interest; be clear about their own values and interests regarding an evaluation; and be honest in what is feasible based on the resources, time, and capacity of the program.

4. Respect for People: Evaluators respect the security, dignity, and self-worth of respondents, program participants, clients, and other evaluation stakeholders. In rural evaluation, contextual factors impact the planning, implementation, and results. Evaluators must be aware of these factors and address them in the evaluation plan. Due to the relatively small population of rural communities, confidentiality is very important.

5. Responsibilities for General and Public Welfare: Evaluators articulate and take into account the diversity of general and public interests and values that may be related to the evaluation. In rural evaluation, it is important to engage stakeholders early in the planning process. When planning and reporting evaluations, evaluators should include relevant perspectives and interests of the full range of stakeholders. Differences and conflicts may arise; rural evaluators should work to resolve these in a professional manner. Finally, evaluators must also keep in mind the public interest and good of all rural populations, not just the group that is involved in a program or intervention.

When we consider these guiding principles, we must consider cultural differences in rural vs. urban evaluation contexts.

How is the culture of rural America different than urban areas?

We know that culture is driven by context, history, values, norms, and economic and political systems. In Chapter 1, we learned about the population of rural America, the history, and some of the unique differences between rural and urban America. The culture within rural America is a blend of race, ethnicity, relation, language, history, sexual orientation, age, and gender. Katherine Clama identified five demographic factors of people who live in rural America. Their behaviors and actions are influenced by these five factors: being older, having less education, living on a farm or in a smaller town, having parents and extended family living in the rural area, and having not travelled far (2004). In rural populations, presentation and body language are also different. In some cases, eye contact or a handshake may be normative, while in other rural cultures, not making eye contact is considered respectful. Some people may prefer more personal space—imagine living in a wide open space without people and then arriving in an office or crowded school. Naturally, the confines of space and people can be overwhelming. In urban communities, riding a subway crammed with people, standing in long lines in close proximity with others is just part of life. This is not the case in rural America.

A changing culture

Culture changes, and because of this, culture is a shifting target for evaluators. Consider how the culture of rural America has changed in the last decade. Rural community members are moving to urban areas for better employment opportunities and access to health care. At the same time, rural America is seeing increases in Native American, Hispanic, and immigrant populations. These groups add to the unique culture of rural America. Therefore, as rural evaluators we must engage in a continual process of being self-aware of our own culture and that of the community or the population that we are working with. Patton acknowledged the importance of culture and the diversity of what we see based on our interests, bias, culture, and values:

> When looking at the same scene, design, object, different people will 'see' different things. What people 'see' is highly dependent on their interests, biases, and backgrounds. Our culture tells us what to see; our early childhood socialization instructs us in how to look at the world; and our value systems tell us how to interpret what passes before our eyes.
>
> *(1999, p. 1199)*

How can evaluators make sure they are culturally competent?

A primary characteristic of culturally competent evaluators is that they recognize the culture, they appreciate the culture, and they incorporate the culture into their evaluation practice (Sen Gupta, Hopson, & Thompson-Robinson, 2004). Guiding principles can help us be more culturally competent in our evaluation approach. A review of guiding principles in cultural competence from community organizing, education, and health care are similar in their recommendations for being culturally competent (Box 3.2).

To begin, evaluators must value and recognize diversity. This requires an understanding and acceptance of differences in cultural backgrounds, communication, values, and ways of knowing. Second, be self-aware. Evaluators have their own culture and values, and because of this, evaluations cannot be value free (Pettifor, 1995). As rural evaluators, our own experiences, skills, values, beliefs, and history actually shape how we conduct evaluations and our relationships in and with communities. Third, know the factors that impact interaction and relationships. Consider the historical experiences of a community in relation to evaluation. Know that across cultures, groups, and within cultures, there is likely a history that contributes to the interactions that you have with the community, as an evaluator. Consider a rural community that has been penalized by an evaluator historically. They may view all evaluators as punitive and not trustworthy. Understanding these histories and other factors that may contribute to relationships with communities is important and driven by culture. Finally,

---

BOX 3.2 Field notes, guiding principles for culturally competent evaluation

1. Value and recognize diversity of rural America.
2. Be self-aware.
3. Know the factors that impact interactions and relationships in rural communities.
4. Integrate cultural knowledge in the evaluation approach.

integrate cultural knowledge in the evaluation approach. Rural evaluators can design evaluations based on an understanding of culture and local knowledge.

Tools for assessing an evaluator's cultural competence

Several tools can help evaluators assess their cultural competence.

The AEA recommends that evaluators plan, implement, and communicate culturally competent evaluation methods (AEA, 2011). From this list, evaluators can examine how often they employ these methods using a 3-point scale, where 1 is never and 3 is always (Table 3.1). This checklist could also be given to stakeholders of a given program, where rural evaluators are working and used as a discussion tool to improve cultural responsiveness. Revisiting these statements often will help rural evaluators attend to culturally appropriate evaluation methods.

TABLE 3.1 Checklist for Culturally Appropriate Evaluation Methods

Statement…	1 = Never 2 = Sometimes 3 = Always
I ensure that the members of the evaluation team collectively demonstrate cultural competence in the context for each evaluation.	
I select or create data collection instruments that have been (or will be) vetted for use with the population of interest.	
I engage in ongoing critical reflection on assumptions about what constitutes meaningful, reliable, and valid data and how these data are derived.	
I employ data collection and analysis methods that address cultural differences in how knowledge is constructed and communicated.	
I use intermediaries to assist with collecting data from persons whose participation would otherwise be limited by language, abilities, or factors such as familiarity or trust.	
I engage and consult with those groups who are the focus of the evaluation in the analysis and interpretation of data, to address multiple audience perspectives.	
I recognize that reporting at different stages of the evaluation may introduce new audiences that can require new culturally appropriate communication strategies.	
I tailor methods of reporting to stakeholder audiences in ways that address issues related to communication and language (may require multiple reports and reporting methods).	
I employ culturally appropriate approaches in the metaevaluation process, including feedback from communities affected by the evaluation.	

Source: Adapted from the AEA Recommendations for Employing Culturally Appropriate Methods (2011).

The Ethnic–Sensitive Inventory was developed by Ho in 1990 to improve social work practitioner's skills for working with ethnic minority clients. This 24-item checklist includes statements like "I realize that my own ethnic and class background may influence my effectiveness" and "I consider it an obligation to familiarize myself with their culture, history, and other ethnically related responses to problems". Practitioners respond to each statement by circling their level of agreement based on a 5-point scale, where 5 is always and 1 is never.

The Culturally Responsive Assessment Tool was developed as a global assessment of culturally responsive practices. Although this is most often used in school settings by teachers, evaluators can learn from this tool. The checklist includes statements related to assessment and accountability, instruction, family and community engagement, professional development, and environment (http://indiana.edu/~pbisin/resources/CRAssessmentCRAprofile12.18.2014.pdf).

Some of the challenges that rural evaluators experience relate to the cultural differences in how evaluators practice evaluation. For example, deficit-based or need-based approaches may not be culturally responsive in rural communities. In other cases, there may be differences in ethics based on culture. Knowing the community and culture first is important for evaluators who work in rural America—especially since the evaluator and the evaluee or community are often from different cultures.

Examples of standards that support cultural competence in evaluation

Culturally and Linguistically Appropriate Services standards

The United States Department of Health and Human Services (USDHHS) Office of Minority Health developed the National Standards for Culturally and Linguistically Appropriate Services (CLAS) in Health and Health Care. CLAS goals are to improve the quality of health care and promote equity in diverse communities. CLAS standards are based on the principle that services are responsive to the cultural health beliefs, practices, preferred language, health literacy, and communication needs of a diverse population or culture (USDHHS Office of Minority Health, ND).

National education association

Schools throughout the country are becoming more diverse. In 1972, just 22% of the public school enrollment were minorities. In 2005, more than 42% of the students enrolled in public schools are from a minority group. More than 10 million students enrolled in public schools throughout the United States speak a language other than English when at home (USDOE, 2007). The National Education Association reports that cultural gaps between teachers and students directly affect their learning outcomes (2007). Rural evaluators can learn from this and ensure that the cultural gaps are bridged, and the language used to communicate information is appropriate for the rural population.

Joint committee on standards for educational evaluation

Beginning in 1975, the Joint Committee on Standards for Educational Evaluation promoted the standards for evaluation professionals that are embraced by most evaluators. These support culturally responsive evaluation and focus on utility, feasibility, propriety, accuracy, and evaluation accountability standards (CDC, 2014). Briefly, *utility* relates to the credibility of the evaluator, the purpose, values, meaning, and information used. *Feasibility* as a culturally competent rural evaluator includes allowing time, being flexible, and understanding the context of rural America. *Propriety* requires inclusiveness and valuing the diversity of the population. *Accuracy* relates to using valid information and terms that have shared meanings. It also requires that stakeholders are part of the evaluation findings process. *Evaluation and accountability standards* in a rural evaluation context ensure that documentation is clear and understandable to all stakeholder groups. It also ensures that everyone that contributed to the evaluation process and product are acknowledged. Last, these standards can be further integrated when persons from the rural community review evaluation findings and reports.

African evaluation association guidelines

African American populations represent a culturally distinct population in rural America. An emerging body of literature points to the importance of evaluation guidelines for working with African American populations. The African Evaluation Association (AfrEA) developed guidelines for evaluators working with African countries, but these guidelines also apply to evaluation in the United States (Hood, 2004. Guidelines were developed in 2006 and based on the Joint Committee on Standards for Education Evaluation (summarized above). Guidelines include 35 standards that are based on four areas: (1) utility for produced information and expected and provided results; (2) feasibility for realism, cautiousness, and efficiency; (3) respect of ethics and respect of legal and ethical rules; and (4) precision and quality for a relevant methodology related to the goal and subject matter of the evaluation (Leslie et al. 2015, para. 4). Hood reports that 30 evaluation standards from AfrEA were adopted as African evaluation guidelines for US evaluators (2004). Cultural considerations were revised in the US standards to reflect rights of human subject, human interactions, and formal agreements (Hood, 2004, p. 34). Rodney Hood is one of the leading authors on culturally responsive evaluation and wrote,

> I have argued that most American evaluation models have not been responsive to less powerful stakeholders in America who are typically members

of racial minorities and / or poor. So why should one assume that American evaluators know what is needed in the context of African educational evaluation?

(p. 33)

Culturally competent resources

There are numerous resources available to rural evaluators. Some of these resources were developed for educators, researchers, or program staff—but cultural competence has several common characteristics across disciplines.

The Culturally Responsive Evaluation and Assessment Resource Center is located at the University of Illinois at Urbana-Champaign in the College of Education and provides resources and support for evaluators as they seek to be culturally responsive (https://crea.education.illinois.edu/). The Culturally Responsive Evaluation and Assessment (CREA) Resource Center supports evaluators, researchers, and communities as they seek to engage in rigorous evaluation and meaningful discussions that support culturally diverse communities.

The Centers for Disease Control developed a resource guide for practicing cultural competence in public health evaluation (CDC, 2014). In rural communities, this resource guide may help focus the evaluation while being more culturally responsive. The Center's for Disease Control (CDC) recommends a six-stage practice for being culturally competent. This begins with engaging stakeholders, describing the program, focusing the evaluation design, gathering credible evidence, justify conclusion, and ensure use and lessons learned (CDC, 2014).

The National Science Foundation's (NSF) Beyond Rigor website includes evaluation resources for working with diverse populations (http://beyondrigor.org/index.html). Seekers will find a variety of practical tips for working with diverse populations, which will help them be more culturally competent. These include tips for accurate data collection, appropriate analysis, context, and recommendations for funding agencies who work with diverse communities.

The NSF is committed to culturally responsive evaluation. NSF developed a handbook for implementing evaluation and addressing cultural responsiveness in evaluation (www.nsf.gov/pubs/2002/nsf02057/nsf02057.pdf). The NSF handbook calls attention to the need for cultural competence in evaluation and how to include culture in all aspects of the evaluation from preplanning to outcomes and disseminating results (Frierson, Hood, & Hughes, 2002). Frierson, Hood, Hughes, and Thomas extended their work on culturally responsive evaluation in their 2010 National Science Foundation User Friendly Guide to Project Evaluation (p. 75):

> Culturally responsive evaluators honor the cultural context in which an evaluation takes place by bringing needed, shared life experiences and

understandings to the evaluation tasks at hand and hearing diverse voices and perspectives. The approach requires that evaluators critically examine culturally relevant but often neglected variables in project design and evaluation. In order to accomplish this task, the evaluator must have a keen awareness of the context in which the project is taking place and an understanding of how this context might influence the behavior of individuals in the project.

The National Center for Cultural Competence at Georgetown University aims to increase the capacity of health care and mental health programs as they design and evaluate culturally and linguistically competent service delivery systems. The National Center recognizes the growing diversity of the US population, persistent disparities, and the need for health equity (https://nccc.georgetown.edu/).

Participatory approaches that support culturally competent evaluation

Community-Based Participatory Research (CBPR) is about a process of equity and action. CBPR is driven by topics that are important to the community. This approach advocates for social change to improve community outcomes (Minkler, Blackwell, Thompson, & Tamir, 2003)—this is practicing cultural competency.

Fisher and Ball's Tribal Participatory Research Model was developed in 2002 for American Indian communities using principles of CBPR. The Tribal Participatory Research (TPR) approach is driven by the culture of a tribe, their social values and kinship systems, and the collaborative process that develops between the evaluator and the community (Fisher & Ball, 2002).

Participatory Culture-Specific Consultation (PCSC) is a participatory approach to evaluation and research that emerged from a dissertation (Varjas, 2003). Since 2003, the PCSC has been used to explore how cultural specificity is integrated into the approach and how the evidence is used to document culturally specific needs and outcomes. The PCSC advocates for negotiation between cross-cultural partners, with ongoing data collection that is continually modified to ensure local cultural fit (Varjas, 2003).

Indigenous Evaluation Framework (IEF) was developed by the American Indian Higher Education Consortium in response to the need to combine Indigenous ways of knowing with Western evaluation approaches. The core values that embody the IEF approach include indigenous knowledge creation and context, people of a place, recognizing our gifts and personal sovereignty, centrality of community and family, and tribal sovereignty (LaFrance & Nichols, 2008).

In addition to these resources, there are several research and evaluation approaches that support culturally responsive evaluation with specific cultures. Let's take a closer look at these.

Case examples with specific cultures in rural America

There are many different cultures in rural America. Evaluators have been working with culturally diverse groups in rural America for a long time; let's read more about ethical challenges, solutions, and approaches for culturally specific evaluation in rural America.

Rural Hispanic populations account for more than 25% of the population growth in rural America (Kandel & Cromartie, 2004). Hispanic is not a racial classification but an ethnic distinction. Rural Hispanic populations may come from Mexico, Central America, and South America. The primary language that Hispanics speak is Spanish. Hispanic cultures have different values, beliefs, and views of the world, that is, they are not all the same. With lower education, limited opportunities for higher paying jobs, and lower educational attainment, Hispanic populations in rural America are considered a vulnerable group (Engstrom, 2017). Conducting program evaluation with Hispanics in rural communities requires an understanding of ethical issues and challenges that may arise. Loi and McDermott called for ethical evaluation in their 2010 article Conducting Program Evaluation with Hispanics in Rural Settings and focused on two areas: (1) informed consent takes into account literacy levels and comprehension, and (2) payment is not considered coercive for participating in a program. Loi and McDermott also stress the importance of building trust (2010). Rural evaluators can overcome trust issues by working with gatekeepers who provide access to the community and ensure ethical evaluation.

Multicultural populations in rural America present a unique challenge for evaluators as they strive for cultural competence. Harris et al. (2007) discuss some of the challenges of evaluating a multicultural school-based intervention in rural Idaho. Student participants involved in the Idaho Consortium for Safe Schools Healthy Students were White, non-Hispanic, Hispanic, Native American, African American, and Asian/Pacific Islander (Harris et al., 2007). Authors report challenges and solutions for multicultural evaluation: (1) it is difficult to implement programs with fidelity when models are not ethnic specific, (2) limited resources, and (3) the need to build trust (2007). Evaluators can overcome these challenges by using participatory evaluation methods and using an evaluation team who is familiar with the culture and setting (Harris et al., 2007). Harris and colleagues (2007) stress the importance of culturally responsive evaluation, "The importance of understanding local conditions and rural sensitivities cannot be underestimated when planning a comprehensive evaluation of school-community initiatives" (p. 89).

Older adults in rural America are a unique, understudied population. Rural older adults experience a lack of affordable transportation, accessible transportation, and social isolation, and are limited with regard to organized activities (Paschoa & Ashton, 2016). Authors Paschoa & Ashton implemented a rural exercise program in the Southeastern United States with women, aged 55–89 years, who were African American, White, and Hispanic (2016). To be culturally responsive to the unique needs or rural older Americans, authors recommend the following: spend time with participants, bring in experts to facilitate discussions, promote the program to increase involvement, add intergenerational participants to address motivation and boredom (Paschoa & Ashton, 2016). While these recommendations are specific to evaluation of physical activity programs, they can also be used in other rural adult program evaluations.

American Indian populations in rural America represent unique histories, geographies, languages, traditions, and values. Authors Bethany Letiecq and Sandra Bailey from Montana State University shared their experience evaluating a five-year US Department of Agriculture Children Youth and Families At-Risk grant (2004). The goal of this grant was to improve the quality and quantity of programs for children, youth, and families through the Extension Service. The evaluation took place on a small reservation of 2,500 people in rural Montana. Through their experience, they wrote about the need to challenge the power differentials and ideas about what good research (and evaluation) looks like (Letiecq & Bailey, 2004). While evaluating the program, they encountered several challenges. The first challenge was the resistance of program staff to participate in the formal evaluation. To overcome this challenge authors invited project staff and community members to identify processes, outcomes, and instruments that would be used in evaluation drawing from utilization-focused evaluation, participatory evaluation, and Fisher and Ball's Tribal Participatory Research Model (all mentioned previously in this chapter). Other challenging factors that the authors discussed were limited resources, appropriate measurement instruments, issues with maintaining confidentiality, logistical constraints due to geographical location, and different ways of knowing. Letiecq and Bailey wrote, "Our majority culture tends to support direct and assertive communication styles when completing tasks, whereas our Native colleagues' cultural milieu supports an outwardly passive style of interaction, particularly among women" (2004, p. 352).

Summary

Cultural competence in evaluation. What does cultural competence really mean? In this chapter, we have touched on some of the definitions and terms, but this is really just the beginning. We learned that culture is constantly changing, and the culture of rural America has changed drastically in the last decade. Our own culture is changing and evolving too. We learned about different culturally competent evaluation approaches that are action based and value driven. In this chapter, we also reviewed various evaluation standards and how they can be used to measure culturally competent evaluation and outcomes. Case examples demonstrated the unique challenges and considerations for rural evaluation with culturally distinct groups. Perhaps the greatest piece of knowledge that you can take away from this chapter is that we are cultural. We are people with histories, values, and even biases that must be acknowledged in our work as rural evaluators. What does your cultural self-assessment say about you?

Points to remember

1. As a rural evaluator, embrace culture and understand how it is incorporated in evaluation.
2. Recognize how dominant systems have marginalized disadvantaged groups in evaluation. Examine your role and relationship with rural communities, and ensure that it promotes equity, collaboration, and community voice.
3. Practice self-awareness, and know your own histories, values, and cultures. Seek involvement from individuals who are part of the culture or familiar with the culture that you are working with.
4. Follow AEA guidelines for culturally competent evaluation and guiding ethics.
5. Use culturally responsive evaluation approaches, and review resources for practicing culturally competent evaluation.
6. Know that culture is fluid and changing, and be aware of these changes and their relation to evaluation.

Additional reading and resources

On Culture in Evaluation
The Colorado Trust Foundation, Retrieved from http://www.communityscience. com/pubs/CrossCulturalGuide.r3.pdf

On Ethics and Principles
AEA's Guiding Principles for Evaluation, http://www.eval.org/p/cm/ld/fid=51

On Culturally Competent Organizations
The Community Tool Box, https://ctb.ku.edu/en/table-of-contents/culture/ cultural-competence/culturally-competent-organizations/main

On Culturally Competent Evaluation
The Centers for Disease Control, https://www.cdc.gov/dhdsp/docs/cultural_ competence_guide.pdf

On African Evaluation Standards
http://afrea.org/

On the Indigenous Evaluation Framework, American Indian Higher Education Consortium
https://portalcentral.aihec.org/indigeval/Pages/default.aspx

Chapter questions

1. Define these terms in your own words: cross-cultural, acculturation, cultural competence, multiculturalism, linguistic competence, and validity. For each definition, provide an example of this term in a rural American community.
2. List the AEA guiding ethics for cultural competence.

3. List the standards of the Joint Committee for Educational Evaluation in a rural cultural context. How might these standards be different in urban areas? How might these standards be similar in both rural and urban areas?
4. Review the guiding principles of culturally competent evaluation. How might you apply these to rural evaluation contexts? Can you think of instances when it would be difficult to apply these principles?
5. Go to the Georgetown University National Center for Cultural Competence website (https://nccc.georgetown.edu/assessments/index.php). Complete one of the online or printed self-assessments. Review your results and summarize how they might apply to rural communities and contexts? How might the focus on culture be different for health-care practitioners compared with evaluators?
6. Summarize the six-step process of the Center for Disease Control for ensuring culturally competent evaluation. For each step, reflect on what this might look like within a rural-focused evaluation and culture.

Practice

1. Go to the Community Toolbox, Chapter 2, Building Relationships with People from Different Cultures (https://ctb.ku.edu/en/table-of-contents/culture/cultural-competence/building-relationships/main). Respond to these two questions: how do you learn about people's cultures, and how do you build relationships with people from other cultures?
2. List the different approaches available that support a culturally competent evaluation approach. How are these similar and how are they different? Can you think of other approaches that support cultural competence in rural America?
3. How many different definitions of culture can you find on the internet? How many definitions of cultural competence can you find? Select the terms that you feel are most appropriate for rural evaluation contexts.

References

Aguado Loi, C., & McDermott, R. (2010) Conducting program evaluation with Hispanics in rural settings. *American Journal of Health Education, 41*(4), 252–256. doi:10.1080/19325037.2010.10599151

American Evaluation Association (2011). *American evaluation association public statement on cultural competence in evaluation.* Fairhaven, MA: Author. Retrieved from http://www.eval.org

American Evaluation Association (2013). *Guiding Principles Review Task Force: Report to the AEA Membership.* Retrieved from https://www.eval.org/p/cm/ld/fid=51

Campbell, P., & Jolly, E. (ND). *Beyond rigor: In a sea of context.* Retrieved from http://beyondrigor.org/PDF/BeyondRigor_InASeaOfContext.pdf

Centers for Disease Control and Prevention (2014). *Practical strategies for culturally competent evaluation.* Atlanta, GA: US Department of Health and Human Services.

Chouinard, J. A., & Cousins, J. B. (2009). A review and synthesis of current research on cross-cultural evaluation. *American Journal of Evaluation, 30*(4), 457–494.

Cultural Responsive Assessment (ND). *Indiana University.* Retrieved from http://indiana.edu/~pbisin/resources/CRAssessmentCRAprofile12.18.2014.pdf

Engstrom, D. (2017). *Hispanics in the United States. An agenda for the twenty-first century.* EBook. Retrieved from https://www.taylorfrancis.com/books/e/9781351515740

Frierson, H. T., Hood, S., & Hughes, G. B. (2002). Strategies that address culturally-responsive evaluation. In J. F. Westat (Ed.), *The 2002 user friendly handbook for project evaluation* (pp. 63–73). Arlington, VA: National Science Foundation. Retrieved from http://www.nsf.gov/pubs/2002/nsf02057/nsf02057.pdf

Georgetown University (2018). *National center for cultural competence. Cultural and linguistic competence health practitioners assessment.* Retrieved from https://www.clchpa.org/

Harris, E., McFarland, J., Siebold, W., Aguilar, R., & Sarmiento, A. (2007). Universal prevention program outcomes. *Journal of School Violence, 6*(2), 75–91. doi:10.1300/J202v06n02_05

Ho, M. K. (1990). Use of ethnic-sensitive inventory (ESI) to enhance practitioner skills with minorities. *Journal of Multicultural Social Work, 1*(1), 57–68.

Hood, S. (2004). A journey to understand the role of culture in program evaluation: Snapshots and personal reflections of one African American evaluator. *New Directions for Evaluation, 2004*(102), 21–37.

Kandel, W., & Cromartie, J. (2004). *New patterns of Hispanic settlement in rural America.* Washington, DC: US Department Agriculture, Economic Research Service. Retrieved from https://pdfs.semanticscholar.org/8afa/903dd4e32e0103b11bcea0955ba8af980332.pdf

Hopson, R. K., & Kirkhart, K. E. (2012). *Strengthening Evaluation Through Cultural Relevance and Cultural Competence.* Workshop presented at the American Evaluation Association/Centers for Disease Control 2012 Summer Evaluation Institute, Atlanta, Georgia, June 2012. Retrieved from http://comm.eval.org/HigherLogic/System/DownloadDocumentFile.ashx?DocumentFileKey=431b5252-b546-445b-aeef-6347b5deeae9.

LaFrance, J., & Nichols, R. (2008). Reframing evaluation: Defining an indigenous evaluation framework. *The Canadian Journal of Program Evaluation, 23*(2), 13.

Leslie, M., Moodley, N., Goldman, I., Jacob, C., Podems, D., Everett, M. et al., (2015). Developing evaluation standards and assessing evaluation quality. *African Evaluation Journal, 3*(1), Art. #112, 13 pages. doi:10.4102/aej.v3i1.112

Letiecq, B., & Bailey, S. (2004). Evaluating from the outside: Conducting cross-cultural evaluation research on an American Indian reservation. *Evaluation Review, 28*(4), 342–357. doi:10.1177/0193841X04265185

Merryfield, M. M. (1985). The challenge of cross-cultural evaluation: Some views from the field. *New Directions for Evaluation, 1985*(25), 3–17.

Mertens, D. (2015). *Research and evaluation in education and psychology.* 4th edition. Thousand Oaks, CA: Sage Publications.

Minkler, M., Blackwell, A. G., Thompson, M., & Tamir, H. (2003). Community-based participatory research: Implications for public health funding. *American Journal of Public Health, 93*(8), 1210–1213.

Paschoa, L., & Ashton, C. (2016). The evaluation of an exercise program for older rural adults. *Activities, Adaptation & Aging, 40*(1), 67–77. doi:10.1080/01924788.2016.1127075

Patton, M. Q. (1999). Enhancing the quality and credibility of qualitative analysis. *Health Services Research, 34*(5 Pt 2), 1189–1208, p. 1199.

Pettifor, J. (1995). Ethics and social justice in program evaluation: Are evaluators value free? *Canadian Journal of School Psychology, 10*, 138–146. doi:10.1177/082957359501000206

SenGupta, S., Hopson, R., & Thompson-Robinson, M. (2004). Cultural competence in evaluation: An overview. *New Directions for Evaluation, 2004*(102), 5–19.

United States Department of Education (2007). *The condition of education.* Washington, DC: The US Department of Education, Institute of Education Sciences. Retrieved from http://nces.ed.gov/program/coe

United States Department of Health and Human Services Office of Minority Health (ND). *The National CLAS Standards.* Retrieved from https://minorityhealth.hhs.gov/omh/browse.aspx?lvl=2&lvlid=53

Varjas, K. M. (2003). *A participatory culture-specific consultation (PCSC) approach to intervention development.* Unpublished doctoral dissertation University at Albany, State University of New York.

4

EVALUATION APPROACHES, MODELS, AND DESIGNS

The secret of getting ahead is getting started. The secret of getting started is breaking your complex overwhelming tasks into management tasks, and then starting on the first one.

–Mark Twain

Evaluation models are like cars: there are different models based on the money you have, the places that you want to go, and the number of seats that you need. Evaluation models can be basic, or extremely complex. The evaluation model you select depends on community's needs, the resources and time available, and the questions that you need answered. Logic models often take a front row seat and give you a visual road map of where you intend to go. Hang on, this is going to be an exciting ride through evaluation models, approaches, and designs.

Selecting an appropriate evaluation model, approach, or design can be difficult in rural communities. Mainly because a lot of designs are tested in urban contexts, at universities or research and evaluation centers with larger populations. The purpose of this chapter is to introduce different evaluation approaches that have been used in rural America. With a basic understanding of the terms model, approach, and design, you will be more comfortable as a rural evaluator.

"Evaluation is a systematic approach for determining the value of something" (AEA, 2014). How do we evaluate in rural communities? Evaluation approaches are a good place to start.

Evaluation approach

An evaluation approach is really about how we begin. There are various approaches rural evaluators use depending on the needs of the community, funding agency, and stakeholders involved. In program evaluation, the approach typically considers factors like program goals, program objectives, funding, and the timeline. Rural evaluators may approach the evaluation through the lens of process, outcome, impact, or economic evaluation. In some cases, other evaluation approaches are used. Since most of these approaches are used in program evaluation, let's review what program evaluation means.

A **program** is a set of resources and activities directed toward one or more common goals (Newcomer, Hatry, & Wholey, 1994). **Program evaluation** is a systematic process of obtaining information to be used to assess and improve a program. Organizations and communities use program evaluations to distinguish successful program efforts from ineffective program activities and services. Results from evaluations can be used to revise existing programs to achieve successful results. Evaluations are a crucial part of any program. When considering the evaluation approach, consider the mission and goals of the program (OVC, 2010).

Hogan (2007) describes six separate approaches used in program evaluation in the 21st century. These are objectives-oriented, management-oriented, consumer-oriented, expertise-oriented, adversary-oriented, and participant-oriented evaluation. Let's take a look at each of these approaches in more detail.

Objectives-oriented evaluation approaches were conceptualized in 1932 by Ralph Tyler (Hogan, 2007). Tyler emphasized the importance of defining goals and objectives in evaluation, and then using these to determine if a program was effective. This approach was criticized because of potential bias in the selection of goals and objectives (Hogan, 2007).

Management-oriented evaluation approaches are most often used by leaders of organizations. Management-oriented approaches are based on context, input, process, and product evaluation (CIPP). A criticism of this approach is that evaluators may be partial to organizational leaders and not be able to respond to evaluation questions early in the process to ensure that a program is delivered as planned. Despite these criticisms, CIPP has been used by internal evaluators, external evaluators, and service providers (Stufflebeam, Madaus, & Kellaghan, 2000).

Consumer-oriented evaluation approaches are often used by governments and consumers to evaluate effectiveness of a product or program (Hogan, 2007). From this approach, formative and summative evaluation emerged. We will review formative and summative evaluation later in this chapter.

Expertise-oriented evaluation approaches are used to determine the value of a program, activity, or institution (Hogan, 2007). Typically, an expertise-oriented approach includes a group of experts who review a program and then make recommendations about that program based on their own experience. A limitation of this approach is that it only includes "experts" and their views may be biased.

Adversary-oriented evaluation approaches are used to uncover results based on opposing views (Hogan, 2007). Typically, an adversarial approach includes judicial proceedings (hearing, prosecution, jury, and defense). This approach brings to light positive and negative aspects of a program, product, or problem. A criticism of this approach is that it seeks to find guilt rather than to improve programs, products, or solve problems.

Participant-oriented evaluation approaches are often used in rural evaluation contexts because they include the experiences of rural community members, stakeholders, and programs as they work together to define what is needed and how to address these needs and evaluate them.

Other 21st-century program evaluation approaches used in rural program evaluation that focus on training are summarized in the next section.

Context Income Reaction and Outcome (CIRO) evaluation approaches are used to evaluate management training including context, input, reactions, and outcomes (Warr, Bird, & Rackham, 1970). CIRO utilizes measures to document knowledge or experience before and after a training (Tennant, Boonkrong, & Roberts, 2002).

Kirkpatrick's evaluation approach was developed in 1959 and includes four types of training outcomes: reactions to training, knowledge or skill acquisition, behavior change, and improvement in individual or organizational outcomes (Hogan, 2007; Kirkpatrick, 1996). The Kirkpatrick evaluation approach is one of the most commonly used evaluation approaches used in training and development.

Phillips's evaluation approach builds on Kirkpatrick's four-level approach and seeks to document the return on investment (ROI) resulting from a training. A benefit of adding ROI to Kirkpatrick's approach is knowing the monetary value of training efforts. A limitation of the ROI is that it can be difficult to enumerate and quantify the complete value.

Success Case Method (SCM) is a process that evaluates both training and strategy. Brinkerhoff describes two primary steps in SCM: (1) survey sample of trainees who attended training and ask, "To what extent have you used your recent training in a way that you believe has made a significant difference to the business?", and (2) identify small groups of trainees who felt the training was successful or unsuccessful. Small groups are interviewed to determine the value of the application and learning, and contextual factors that helped trainees use training (2005, p. 93). SCM results in in-depth narratives about the effect on business and knowledge about the factors that improve or impede training (Brinkerhoff, 2005).

Evaluation approaches frequently used in rural communities

Monitoring evaluation (ME) is used in rural evaluation contexts when the evaluation seeks to document program plans and directions, to determine if the program is on task and on track to meet deadlines and goals. There are three approaches to ME, component analysis, developed performance assessment, and systems analysis (Owen, 2007). The goal of ME is to improve delivery, reach, outcomes, or processes. Indicators that are used in ME may include appropriateness, efficiency, and effectiveness (Owen, 2007). Using these indicators as a guide, evaluators can support rural communities by providing useful feedback on how programs are being managed and implemented. ME is useful for evidence-based policy making with a focus on impact and results (Gertler, Martinez, Premand, Rawlings, & Vermeersch, 2016). For more information on ME, review the resources section at the end of this chapter.

Participatory/collaborative evaluation emphasizes participatory/collaborative forms of evaluation, and engaging stakeholders in the evaluation process. This helps stakeholders understand evaluation and the program being evaluated, and ultimately uses the evaluation findings for decision-making purposes. As with utilization-focused evaluation (UFE), the primary question guiding participatory evaluation is, "What are the information needs of those closest to the program?" These needs are then incorporated into the evaluation design and revisited throughout the evaluation process (Cousins & Earl, 1995).

Rapid Rural Appraisal (RRA). This collaborative approach was developed in the 1980s and was the basis for **Participatory Rural Appraisal (PRA)**. RRA is focused on data collection by outsiders (Chambers, 1994). In the 1990s, **PRA** methods further evolved. Chambers defines PRA as, "an approach and method for learning about rural life and conditions from, with and by rural people" (2005, p. 1). PRA is a process of collaboration, appraisal, and analysis undertaken by community and evaluators. PRA was developed because traditional surveys did not produce quality data about local priorities among developing countries and farmers. An example of PRA is a Venn diagram that documents the importance of agricultural issues, new ideas, and partners (Chambers, 1994). Both approaches have been used in developing countries and are appropriate for rural American evaluation.

Cluster evaluation was developed by the W.K. Kellogg Foundation in 1989. According to Barley & Jenness, "Cluster evaluation involves a skilled and credible evaluator who works with a cluster of projects to assure that useful and defensible information is obtained" (1993, p. 142). This method is useful for strengthening the evaluation approach in rural communities when programs are similar in purpose and scope.

Evaluability assessment is a form of research used to assess the kinds of information that may result from evaluation, the feasibility of the evaluation, and the match of the evaluation with demand (Wholey, 2004). Evaluability assessment begins in the planning stage of evaluation to clarify the goals and design of a program. According to Wholey, there are six key steps in evaluability assessment: involve users, clarify program, explore program, reach agreement, explore alternative designs, and agree on evaluation priorities (Wholey, 2004, p. 36).

Objectives-based impact evaluation is a type of impact evaluation used in rural communities. Concepts of objectives-based evaluation focuses on determining if the goals or objectives of a program have been achieved (Owen, 2007).

Empowerment evaluation is designed to increase the capacity of stakeholders to conduct evaluation (Wandersman et al., 2004). David Fetterman developed empowerment evaluation based on known evaluation concepts, techniques, and results, with the idea that, through this process, conditions could improve, and community members would be empowered to take control of a program or intervention (Fetterman, 2001). Empowerment evaluation requires participation from community, and unlike participatory evaluation approaches, empowerment evaluation is about increasing not only participation of community but their capacity and empowerment. Empowerment evaluation focuses on processes that lead to improvements both in community conditions and programs, and self-determination (Fetterman, 2001). In rural communities, empowerment evaluation approaches are preferred. With limited resources available and emerging evaluation capacity, empowerment evaluation supports developing evaluation skills, tools, and processes that improve outcomes and help communities achieve their goals.

UFE was developed by Michael Quinn Patton for program evaluation (1997). UFE supports evaluators as they facilitate learning and application of evaluation results in real-world contexts. UFE is a guide rather than an evaluation method that can be used alone, or in conjunction with other evaluation approaches and designs. The real benefit of UFE in rural communities is the establishment of capacity for evaluation in a community and the translation of this capacity and knowledge to other programs. Rural evaluation approaches may be more responsive to the needs of the community when they engage stakeholders in all phases of the evaluation process. UFE is one approach that helps ensure their engagement and use of findings.

Theory-driven evaluation is based on the idea that the evaluation comes from a program theory, with explanations for what causes observed outcomes (Donaldson, 2007). Rural programs may benefit from a theory driven evaluation approach because they inform the entire evaluation process. Evaluators facilitate a process of knowing what is supposed to happen as a result of a program or intervention, and what actually happens. Theory-driven evaluation encompasses a large body of knowledge that includes community knowledge, community context, existing theories, and research to design, implement, and analyze evaluation results.

Informal and formal evaluation. The terms informal and formal are used to describe categories of evaluation. Formal evaluations are often characterized by planned activities, prescribed protocols, protection of information, objective scores of measurement, narrowed scope, controlled settings, and strong inferences (Williams & Suen, 1998). In contrast, informal evaluations are often spontaneous, flexible in procedures and protocols, highlight the depth of information available, utilize subjective vs. objective approaches, are subjectively biased, occur in natural or uncontrolled settings, and make broad inferences. Rural community evaluation may be more effective if informal evaluation processes are followed. This allows for greater flexibility which is often required in rural/remote/isolated locations.

There are several different ways to approach an evaluation. The approach and evaluation design may include randomized evaluations, matching methods, regression discontinuity, distributional impacts, and structural modeling approaches (Khandker, Koolwal, & Samad, 2010). These approaches should be selected based on the purpose, time, capacity, and needs of the program. In sum, the goal in rural community evaluation is not to force an approach or protocol on a community but rather to work with the community to design evaluations that support what community members, leaders, and stakeholders want that also meets the funding agency needs.

Table 4.1 outlines common evaluation approaches used in rural America, their purpose, guiding questions, and timing.

TABLE 4.1 Defining Evaluation Purpose, Questions, and Timing

	Purpose	Questions	Timing
Formative evaluation Performance monitoring	Accountability, monitors resource use, documents progress and manages problems that occur.	Have activities been conducted as planned? Have services been offered as a result of the program? Has the effort accomplished what it intended?	When new program is developed. When modifications have been made to an existing program. As needed.
Process evaluation Program monitoring	Understanding about if program is being implemented as planned and on schedule. Documents if program is producing intended outputs. Identifies strengths and weaknesses. Provides critical information for making program modifications.	Has the strategy been implemented as planned, why or why not? What has worked? Why or why not? What needs to be improved now?	Beginning and during implementation.
Outcome evaluation Summative evaluation	Determines if desired outcomes were achieved. Documents what made program effective or ineffective. Explores likelihood that program can be sustained and replicated.	What changes did the program cause? How did the program contribute to these changes? How is the effort going to be sustained and replicated?	After program implementation begins, when program is stable.
Impact evaluation	Review of how program affects outcomes, both positive and negative. Determines if affects are intended or unintended. Helps establish accountability. Contributes to lessons learned. Requires counterfactual of what outcomes would be without a program.	What is the overall impact of the program? What is the nature of impacts and their reach? What influence did other factors have on the impacts? How did the program contribute to impacts? Are impacts sustainable? How? Did the impacts match the needs of the target population?	After the program has been implemented and there is sufficient data to answer impact questions and document impact.

Assessment	Documents understanding. Used to monitor how program is being implemented. A needs assessment is a common tool used in evaluation.	What is known? What is needed? What has changed? What needs to change?	Can be used before and after a program, to make changes, or to inform program strategy and direction. Use of assessment is to monitor how the program is being implemented and make changes to improve process and outcomes.
Economic evaluation Cost analysis Cost-benefit analysis Cost-effectiveness evaluation	Determine the costs of a program. Reduce costs of a program. Monitor program effectiveness related to costs. Supports policy and decision-making. Supports process and impact evaluation findings.	What are the total program costs? What are the cost savings that resulted from the program (health, environment, human life, other)? What is the next cost?	At the beginning of a program. During a program. After a program has been implemented and sufficient cost and outcome data are available to document cost savings from program delivery.

Process and formative evaluation

Process evaluation focuses on implementation of programs using empirical data to assess the delivery of programs (Scheirer, 1994). Its goal is to provide feedback to program leaders, policy makers, and funding agencies. The terms formative and process evaluation are often used interchangeably, but some would argue that formative evaluation is documenting immediate changes when the program is being implemented, whereas process evaluation occurs after there is sufficient information to document what is happening, what is working, and what needs to be improved. **Formative evaluation** occurs when a program is being implemented with the goal of making immediate changes based on recommendations from the evaluation. Sometimes the terms formative evaluation and performance monitoring are used in evaluation. **Performance monitoring** helps support communities as they work toward their goals and implement objectives. Evaluators use process evaluation, formative evaluation, and performance monitoring to support communities as they implement programs. Documentation of the process helps identify areas that can be improved so that a community reaches their goals. But how do rural evaluators begin to design a process evaluation?

Designing a process evaluation

Designing a process evaluation is essential because it the first step in documenting progress and supporting continuous feedback. Saunders, Evans, and Joshi identified six steps for developing a process evaluation plan for health programs (2005). Not all rural program evaluations are health focused, but these steps can help guide evaluators as they work in community to develop process evaluations that work.

1. Describe the program
2. Describe how the program will be delivered
3. Develop potential questions
4. Determine methods
5. Consider program resources, context, and characteristics
6. Finalize the process evaluation plan.

(Saunders, Evans, & Joshin, 2005)

Process evaluation designs support broad objectives; these were identified by Stufflebeam and Shinkfield in 1985 as to:

1. provide feedback about the program activities, expected activities, and delivery of activities to the intended audience;
2. assess the extent to which the program staff carried out their roles and developed partnerships with other organizations; and
3. provide a record of what happened and what happened compared with what was planned.

Impact and outcome evaluation

Impact Evaluation is used to assess impacts in rural programs and interventions. Impact evaluations are critical in rural America because they help us understand outcomes related to a program or intervention. Impact evaluations are concerned with the cause and effect of a given program or intervention and may use a specific formula (Box 4.1).

Impact evaluations can either take place at the beginning, that is, when a program is being designed or after the program has been implemented (Gertler et al., 2016). In rural communities, impact evaluations that occur during the beginning of the program or intervention may be more realistic because they document baseline data and information before any programming or intervention takes place. Sometimes, the effects of a program or intervention are difficult to measure, and collecting baseline impact evaluation data will help you demonstrate the value and impacts of a program.

The time that it takes to conduct an impact evaluation varies, although if you are planning to collect primary data, plan on 18 months. If you are using secondary data in the impact evaluation, it may be possible to conduct an impact evaluation in 12 months (Organization for Economic Co-operation and Development, 2018).

Challenges that rural evaluators encounter when planning and implementing an impact evaluation are numerous. The lack of traditional baseline data or control group is a common problem. In many rural communities, new program funding is granted to explore something that has not been done before. This means that evaluators need to be creative in how they design impact evaluations and identify baseline or control group data. Another impact evaluation challenge is making sure that you have a representative sample—many rural communities have a large land base and trying to reach a sufficient number of people who meet the characteristics and eligibility of a given program or intervention can be difficult. Finding a comparison group that can be used to evaluate the impact of intervention efforts is difficult as well. The last challenge of impact evaluation relates to limited administrative data to demonstrate costs of a program/intervention.

Because impact evaluation can be difficult in rural communities due to limited resources, a small sample, and lack of a control group, we will take a look at how to apply these principles in rural evaluation practice (Box 4.2).

BOX 4.1 Impact evaluation formula

$\Delta = (Y \mid P = 1) - (Y \mid P = 0)$
Δ = Causal Impact of Program(P) on outcome(Y)

BOX 4.2 Principles of impact evaluation in practice

Five Criteria for Impact Evaluation in Rural Communities

#1 Relevance—Were objectives of the intervention/program in-line with the funding agency requirements, community needs, local priorities, and rural policies?

#2 Effectiveness—Were the objectives of the intervention achieved?

#3 Efficiency—Were funds, time, expertise, skills and other resources used to produce results?

#4 Impact—What are the positive and negative impacts produced by the intervention/program that are both intended and unintended? Are there consequences of these impacts that must be addressed?

#5 Sustainability—How will the community continue to benefit after intervention/programming has ended? Is there evidence that the program/ intervention is sustainable?

Source: Adapted from the Organization for Economic
Co-operation and Development (2018)

Impact evaluations are characterized by innovative study designs, pilot programs, and interventions that produce solid evidence (Khandker et al., 2010). **Targets and benchmarks** are indicators used to specify a value of what is to be achieved by a given time. An example of a target in rural evaluation is the number of community town hall meetings that will occur in the first year. **Indicators** document different aspects of the program/intervention outlined in the logic model. **Impact indicators** measure the distal outcomes that occur over time. **Measures** may relate to healthy, well-being, quality of life, poverty, policy, and environment. Measures are defined in the evaluation plan and used to document progress toward goals and objectives. **Monitoring** is different from impact evaluation, and it seeks to evaluate the performance of a program or intervention (Khandker et al., 2010). Sometimes, the terms Monitoring & Evaluation (M&E) are used in evaluation, but the purpose of monitoring compared with evaluation is different.

Outcome evaluation is similar to impact evaluation, but focuses on whether a program or intervention produced the intended results. Logic models can be helpful in conceptualizing outcomes that are short term, intermediate, and long term. Outcome evaluations may include an assessment from the impact evaluation on each program or intervention, data from the population or group involved, and an appropriate evaluation design. When planning an outcome evaluation, it is important to identify the indicators, data, and collection strategy.

Why outcome evaluation?

We can assess the effect of a program using outcome evaluation. Outcome evaluation seeks to show a causal relationship between the program and outcome. To achieve this, an evaluator must first show that the cause (program) came before the effect (outcome). Second, evaluators must show that the cause and effect are related to each other, and that the effect was not caused by something else (Bureau of Justice Assistance Center, 2011).

Planning for the outcome and impact evaluation occurs early in the program period. For many programs, it begins with selecting a study design and developing a logic model. These planning efforts are typically driven by a theory of change. Theory of Change is an explanation of how change happens in a given context (Hearn, 2015). Outcome evaluations are driven by what has changed as a result of the program. With this in mind, in the next section, we will review short-term, intermediate, and long-term outcomes.

Short-term outcomes may be related to knowledge, skills, or attitudes. Short-term outcomes are general measured immediately after the program ends. An example of a short-term outcome is a youth reporting increased knowledge about the dangers of binge drinking. **Intermediate outcomes** are changes in behavior or decision-making that are measured after the program ends. Intermediate and medium-term outcomes are usually measured several months after a program ends. An example of a medium-term outcome is a reduction in the number of underage youth who report no binge drinking in the past 30 days. **Long-term outcomes** are changes in status or life conditions. These are measured over a period of years or several years after the program or intervention has taken place. An example of a long-term outcome is reducing the binge drinking rate in underage youth in a community after an intervention.

What is the difference between outcome and impact evaluation?

Outcome evaluations are used to measure the program effects on the targeted outcome. **Impact** evaluations require a counterfactual description of what would have happened if there were not a program implemented. Impact evaluations build a strong evidence base while providing guidance for future programming and policy. The primary difference between impact and outcome evaluation is the time it takes to document a result: impact evaluation is immediate, whereas outcome evaluation focuses on the long-term results of a program.

Performance monitoring

Most federal agencies have specific evaluation and performance monitoring tasks for rural evaluators. Often these tasks are described as data collection and performance measurement. Performance measures may include the number of people involved in a program or activity related to the goals of the program, the number of organizations involved, the number of individuals screened or referred, the number of people receiving services, and the number or percentage of work group who are part of the community or target population. These performance measures are collected using a standard tool and may be reported daily, monthly, or biannually. Data are used by the funding agencies to document outcomes related to the program and justify funding to congress or other decision makers (Substance Abuse and Mental Health Services Administration, 2017).

Performance assessment

Local performance assessment is also required by most federally funded programs and is designed by the rural evaluator and community, and used to track progress toward program goals, objectives, and outcomes. Local performance assessment uses outcome and process questions. Outcome questions in local performance assessment may include "How has the program impacted the target population?", "Did some elements of the program have a greater impact than others?", "What were the behavior outcomes?", "What were the factors associated with outcomes including race, ethnicity, sexual orientation, and gender identity?", and "How durable were the effects?" (SAMHSA, 2017).

Assessment is similar to evaluation, but focuses more on understanding the process that is being implemented through a series of objective measurements and observations. In contrast, evaluation is about determining the value of something. Assessment is ongoing—it never really ends, whereas evaluation has a beginning and an end. Educators often use assessment to improve a process with a focus on learning, teaching, and outcomes.

Process questions in performance assessment

Process questions used in local performance assessment should be tailored to the community context, culture, program goals, and objectives. Examples of process-related questions include "How closely did the implementation match the plan?", "What changes were made to the original plan and why?", "How did the program address disparities in outcomes across subpopulations including the Culturally and Linguistically Appropriate Services (CLAS) standards?", "Who provides services to whom, in what context, and at what costs?", "How was fidelity assessed overtime?", and "How many individuals were reached through the program?" (SAMHSA, 2017).

Economic evaluation

Economic evaluations are used to determine the economic benefit of a program or intervention while informing public policy. However, economic evaluations are not conducted in a systematic way or integrated into most federal, state, and local programs. The lack of consistent economic evaluation across programs and communities in the United States has resulted in a lack of evidence about what constitutes cost-effectiveness (Grosse, Teutsch, & Haddix, 2007).

Economic evaluations are critical in rural communities because resources are often scarce, and policy makers often want to know what types of programming and interventions will have the greatest impact on cost savings. Economic evaluations can also be used to document cost and find ways to reduce program and intervention costs (CDC, 1995). Other uses include monitoring, recording, or evaluating program effectiveness with a focus on program costs and informing decision makers about costs and outcomes.

Before you begin an economic evaluation, consider these questions: "Who wants to know?", "How will the information be used?", and "Is there sufficient data?". When designing an economic evaluation, it is important to first justify the study. This justification includes the research questions that will be answered in the economic evaluation, the analytical approach, the comparison group, and the approach to costs and outcomes (Fox-Rushby & Cairns, 2005). There are seven primary considerations for economic evaluation, Box 4.3.

Let's review each of these considerations in more detail.

Objectives of analysis relate to what you plan to study or evaluate. **Audience** for the economic evaluation include those who will use the information to make decisions. **Viewpoints** are the perspectives used to examine the costs, the outcomes, and their value. Viewpoints are typically a society's viewpoint, which is a broad perspective of the costs and benefits. In contrast, decision maker viewpoints are narrowly focused to document specific program economic impacts on a desired outcome (Fox-Rushby & Cairns, 2005). **Analytic horizon** is a period of time covering **main** costs and benefits, seasonal or cyclical variations, and the time period of the intervention.

BOX 4.3 Considerations for economic evaluations

Seven Considerations for Economic Evaluation

#1 Objectives of Analysis
#2 Audience
#3 Viewpoints
#4 Period of Time Covered
#5 Intervention
#6 Alternative Intervention/ Comparison Group
#7 Target Population

Source: Fox-Rushby, J. A., & Cairns, J. (2005)

Intervention descriptions must be included in the economic evaluation plan as well. Recommendations for describing interventions in the economic evaluation plan include answering these questions: who does what, to whom, where, how often, and what are the results (Drummond & McGuire, 2001)? **Alternative Intervention/Comparison Groups** are used to calculate effectiveness of intervention and cost savings resulting from an intervention. There are several types of comparison groups that may be used in economic evaluation: single or mixed intervention, best available alternative, group with no intervention or treatment, and different levels of intensity for the intervention. **Target Population** includes age, sex, disease, and geography/rural location.

Formulas for calculating economic impact

Cost analysis is a form of economic evaluation that includes the systematic collection and classification of program costs (Dunet, 2012). **Cost–benefit analysis** (CBA) is measuring costs and benefits of an intervention to determine the costs and consequences of a program or intervention in monetary terms (Robinson, 1993). **Cost-effectiveness** analysis is used to measure the monetary costs and outcomes of a program (Phelps & Mushlin, 1991). **Cost utility** analysis builds on cost-effectiveness analysis but includes both qualitative and quantitative units of measure. One example is using quality-adjusted live years as a health outcome (Dunet, 2012).

The most common economic evaluation used in rural evaluation is a cost analysis or a CBA. CBA is used by rural evaluators to assess the benefits and weaknesses of a given program, policy, or intervention. CBA is also used to determine what approach(es) are needed to achieve the greatest societal benefit. Five steps guide the CBA process: (1) determine the impact, (2) determine whose perspective (society or decision maker), (3) measure the costs, (4) measure the benefits in monetary terms, and (5) compare the costs and benefits (Box 4.4).

There are different types of costs used in CBA. **Variable costs** are those that vary and may include staff time, supplies, materials, lab tests, participant time, and participant expenses. **Fixed costs** are typically known before an intervention and do not vary; these may include promotional materials, facilities rental, equipment, maintenance, administrative and support staff, travel, professional development, and others (CDC, 1995). Formulas for calculating CBA will vary based on the type of program that is being evaluated. The total cost of a program is calculated by adding the total variable costs and the total fixed costs together. To calculate the variable costs, multiply the unit cost of each variable and the total quantity. To calculate the fixed cost, multiply the unit of cost of each fixed input by the quantity and add over all fixed inputs used (CDC, 1995). For more information on economic evaluation and calculating costs, check out the resources section at the end of this chapter.

BOX 4.4 Field notes on CBA

Substance use disorders cost society more than $510.8 billion annually. These losses include lost wages, premature death, injury, incarceration, and decreased quality of life. The Substance Abuse and Mental Health Administration developed a CBA ratio for calculating costs benefits or recovery programs. This ratio is based on a 12:1 impact, meaning that for every dollar spent on the recovery program, the return to society is 12 dollars. The unit cost of the program was and $775.

Determine the impact: we wanted to document the cost savings of peer recovery support.

Determine whose perspective (society or decision maker): we used societal perspectives encompassing crime and criminal justice, health care, and recovery capital.

Measure the costs: we examined the costs of providing peer recovery support and calculated unit costs of $775 per person.

Measure the benefits in monetary terms: we examined cost savings using criminal justice/crime involvement, health-care costs, and recovery capital (education, employment, stable housing, family and community involvement, and life meaning).

Compare the costs and benefits: our program provided recovery support for 206 people between 2014 and 2016. The cost saving based on the 12:1 ratio was $1,915,800.

The basic formula for calculating cost benefit is as follows:

$$\text{Cost}(\text{program or intervention}) + \text{Cost}(\text{side effects})$$
$$- \text{Cost}(\text{health or other outcome averted})$$

Evaluation model

The term **evaluation model** refers to something that can be followed and explained in a systematic way. Often models are visual, describing critical information and how events occur in time and the impact they have. One of the most common models used in evaluation is the logic model.

Logic models

Logic models have been used since the 1970s as a way of telling a story of how a program will work (Bickman, 1987; McLaughlin & Jordan, 1999). Logic models include several elements including context, inputs, activities, outputs, initial outcomes, intermediate outcomes, and long term outcomes (Figure 4.1). Evaluators in rural communities are often asked to develop a logic model, present it to community members and stakeholders, and then make revisions based on

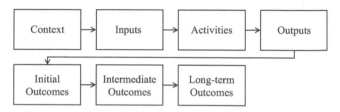

FIGURE 4.1 Logic Model.

feedback received before submitting it to a funding agency for approval. Logic models may be required in the grant application process or they can be used to facilitate monitoring and evaluation once a program is funded. There are many different ways to develop a logic model, Figure 4.1 is just one.

When developing a logic model, here are some definitions to keep in mind:

- Context: This includes the target population, their needs, and the situation that is being addressed through the program/evaluation.
- Inputs: Human, financial, organizational, and community resources needed.
- Activities: What the program does with the inputs. May include processes, events, and actions.
- Outputs: A direct result of the program activities, for example, the number of classes taught.
- Initial outcomes: The changes that resulted from the program, for example, increases in healthy coping skills.
- Intermediate outcomes: Changes in behavior as a result of the program, for example, high school youth choose meditation as a coping strategy.
- Long-term outcomes: The long-term results of the program, for example, improved five-year graduation rates among high school students.

Logic models are needed in rural evaluation contexts to outline a program and articulate underlying assumptions about a theory being used in the evaluation. Previous literature has identified logic models as a theory of action that demonstrates how stakeholders think the program will work (Savaya & Waysman, 2005). As rural evaluators, it is important to work with stakeholders early in the evaluation process to develop a logic model. Revisiting the logic model and updating elements as the program is implemented may be necessary. According to Kaplan and Garret (2005), "Part of the difficulty of logic model development may also be its greatest strength: that it forces planners and managers to think of their projects in a conceptually different way. In its essence, use of the logic model guides program participants in applying the scientific method—the articulation of a clear hypothesis or objective to be tested—to their project development, implementation, and monitoring". (p. 171)

Logic models are appealing because they offer a visual depiction of a process. There are several tools available for developing a logic model. Microsoft Smart

Art is one of the many programs available. Art and drawings that come from the community can also be useful. Storyboards can be helpful when engaging youth, families, and community members in the building of a logic model. We will talk more about visual data sources in Chapter 6.

Outcome sequence chart

At times, it is helpful to focus on a specific part of the logic model. Figure 4.2 is an outcome sequence chart that was developed from a program logic model. This focuses on intermediate outcomes, end outcomes, outputs, and indicators.

For more information on logic models, review Appendix A and the additional resources section at the end of this chapter.

Evaluation design

The evaluation design is based on program goals, research questions, evaluation purpose, and resources available. This section introduces four of the most common evaluation designs (also called methods): experimental, quasi-experimental, nonexperimental, and mixed-methods designs (Figure 4.3).

Experimental designs are considered the most powerful way to determine the causes and effects of a given program. Experimental designs require the randomization of participants into a treatment and a control group. The second most common is a quasi-experimental design. This is similar to the experimental design but does not have random assignment. **Quasi-experimental designs** are most useful when evaluators want to document the effect of a treatment, policy, or intervention. **Nonexperimental designs** may include

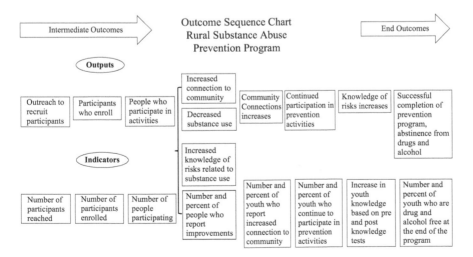

FIGURE 4.2 Prevention Program Outcome Chart.

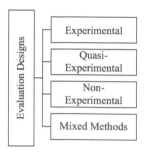

FIGURE 4.3 Evaluation Designs.

pre- and post-intervention studies, case study approaches, and post-intervention approaches. Nonexperimental designs are useful for evaluators in developing program findings, best practices, and improving performance. A limitation of the nonexperimental design is the lack of control of external factors that may influence outcomes.

Mixed-methods designs are increasingly being used in rural evaluation contexts. Greene, Caracelli, and Graham define mixed methods as "those that include at least one quantitative method (designed to collect numbers) and one qualitative method (designed to collect words), where neither type of method is inherently linked to any particular inquiry paradigm" (1989, p. 256).

Basic mixed-methods designs are classified as convergent parallel designs, explanatory sequential designs, or exploratory sequential designs (Creswell, 2013). These designs are similar because they use both qualitative and quantitative data. They are different in how they use data that leads to evaluation results. For example, the convergent parallel design combines qualitative and quantitative data, merges data, and then interprets or explains the convergence or divergence of data based on findings. Explanatory sequential designs use qualitative results to inform quantitative results. Exploratory sequential designs use qualitative data to create results, develop interventions, and instruments to evaluate interventions.

In rural evaluation, mixed-methods designs and nonexperimental designs are common. These designs include one-shot designs, retrospective pretest designs, one group pretest and posttest design, and case study designs. The following are examples of how mixed-methods and nonexperimental designs have been used in rural contexts (Box 4.5).

A final note on these designs. The one-shot design involves gathering information after a program, intervention, or activity. Retrospective pretests are similar to one-shot designs, but ask participants to recall behaviors or conditions that were present before and after. The one-group pretest–posttest design involves collecting data after a program, intervention, or activity. Case study designs are often qualitative in nature and designed to further understanding about the process, context, or systems involved in a program (Preskill & Russ-Eft, 2004).

BOX 4.5 Field notes on evaluation designs in rural practice

One-shot design: we worked with the local high school to implement a suicide prevention training. After the training, we administered a survey to collect data on the knowledge gained, satisfaction, and recommendations for future trainings.

Retrospective pretest: our program is designed to prevent substance use in at-risk youth living in rural Wyoming. Youth attended prevention activities over a six-week period. At the end of the program, youth completed a survey that asked them questions about substance use before and after the program. The information they provided was based on their recollection of their behaviors before and after the program occurred.

One-group pre- and posttest: we developed a job training program for unemployed workers living in a rural Montana community. Before the job training program began, we collected information about their knowledge, skills, and interests. At the end of the training, we collected the same information. We compared these data to learn more about the impact of the job training program.

Case Study: understanding the action planning process in rural communities is important for designing prevention and intervention programming. We designed a case study to understand more about the rural community context, rural community member perspectives, and their experiences as members of the action planning team. Because generalization was not our goal, we focused on qualitative data collection and analyses. These data allowed us to describe the individuals involved, the process in which action planning takes place, and how different organizations and policy makers support or hinder the action planning process. The primary question our action planning case study sought to answer was, "How does the action planning process work in this rural community?"

Research and evaluation

What is the difference?

As evaluators and or researchers, we walk a fine line between **evaluation research**, program evaluation, and **basic research**. Throughout this text, you might notice the terms research and evaluation are used in the same paragraph. The Office of Program Analysis and Evaluation at the National Institute of General Medical Sciences describes the differences between research and evaluation (Table 4.2).

Research is the systematic investigation used to generate facts, test theories, or draw new conclusions about a particular subject (Merriam-Webster, ND). Michael Quinn Patton described the differences between research and evaluation

TABLE 4.2 Differences in Research and Evaluation

Research vs. Evaluation	
Produces generalizable knowledge	Judges merit or worth
Utilizes scientific inquiry based on intellectual curiosity	Utilizes program interests of stakeholder's first
Advances knowledge and theory	Provides information that is used to inform program decision-making
Takes place in a controlled setting	Takes place in various places, with different people, resources, needs, and timelines
Results are published	Results are reported to stakeholders

Source: Blome (2009).

(as cited in 2008 by Sandra Mathison in Fundamental Issues in Evaluation) as the following.

> The difference between research and evaluation, like most of the distinctions we make, perhaps all of them, is arbitrary. One can make the case that the two are the same, or different, along a continuum or on difference continua complete.
>
> *(p. 187)*

Mathison continues the conversation about what distinguishes evaluation and research:

> Evaluation particularizes, research generalizes.
> Evaluation is designed to improve something, research is designed to prove something.
> Evaluation provides the basis for decision making, research provides the basis for conclusions.
> Evaluation is the, "So what?" and Research is the, "What is so?"
> Evaluation is about how well something works. Research is about how it works.
> Evaluation is about value; research is about what is.
>
> *(2008, p. 189)*

Evaluation research is a process of "supplying valid and reliable evidence.... About how programs are planned, how well they operate, and how effectively they achieve their goals" (Monette, Sullivan, & DeJong, 1990, p. 337). In contrast, we know that **program evaluation** is done to provide feedback about what services to provide, to who, and how to provide them most effectively (Zechmeister, Shaughnessy, & Zechmeister, 1996). The evaluation design will depend on the purpose of the evaluation.

You might be wondering if it is necessary to have all three of these, a model, an approach, and a design, in your evaluation plan. The simple answer is, it depends, but generally no. As a rural evaluator you will know what needs to be

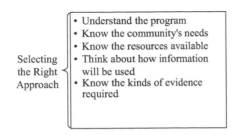

FIGURE 4.4 Selecting the Right Evaluation Approach.

done based on the context, evaluation goals, questions that need to be answered, and the time and funding available. Let's examine some approaches, models, and designs used in rural evaluation contexts.

Selecting the right approach for rural evaluation

With so many designs, models, and approaches, you might be wondering how to select the right one. First you must understand the program. This means understanding what the program intends to accomplish or change and the theory that is underpinning the program and change. It is also good to know the community's needs and how they relate to the program goals and objectives. Sometimes, there are limited resources available in rural communities, so know what resources are available to support the evaluation. Before you select an evaluation design, model, or approach, consider how the information will be used. Imagine the report that you write at the end of the program or intervention. What does the community want to know? What does the funding agency want to know? How can the evaluation help support this end goal? Last, consider the evidence (data) that is required to demonstrate the impacts of the program or intervention. How much time do you have? How many people will participate? Are there sufficient resources available to support? (Figure 4.4).

Summary

This chapter began with an overview of 21st-century program evaluation models and approaches. We reviewed logic models and their use in rural evaluation contexts. This chapter also outlined evaluation designs, how they are selected, and when they are used. Knowing the difference between research and evaluation will help rural evaluators as they seek to find value and worth, and inform decision makers.

Points to remember

1. Evaluation is about finding value, merit, or worth.
2. Research is about building an evidence base, testing or revising theories, and generalizing results.

3. For each evaluation approach, there is a purpose, question, and timing that must be considered in rural evaluation contexts.
4. There are multiple evaluation approaches, designs, and models that can be used in rural evaluation contexts—begin planning the evaluation early and seek involvement from rural stakeholders.
5. Participatory-oriented evaluation approaches are recommended in rural evaluation contexts. These approaches can be blended with other approaches and evaluation designs for maximum impact and utility.

Additional reading and resources

On Empowerment Evaluation
Fetterman, F. (2007). *Empowerment Evaluation*. Retrieved from http://info. davidfetterman.com/documents/EEPresidaddress.pdf

On Evaluation
Green, J., & South, J. (2006). *Evaluation: evaluation*. New York, NY: McGraw Hill International Ltd. Retrieved from https://ebookcentral-proquest-com. libproxy.uncg.edu

On Storyboards and Logic Models
Action Evaluation Collaborative. (ND). *Storyboard Activity*. Retrieved from http://www.betterevaluation.org/en/resources/storyboard_activity

On Impact Evaluation Designs
Khandker, S. R., Koolwal, G. B., & Samad, H. A. (2010). *Handbook on impact evaluation: Quantitative methods and practices*. Washington, DC: World Bank.

On Utilization Focused Evaluation
Patton, M. (2008). *Utilization Focused Evaluation*, 4th edition. Thousand Oaks: Sage Publications.

On Theory Driven Evaluation
Chen, H. T. (1990). *Theory-driven evaluations*. Sage.

On Research vs. Evaluation
Mathison, S. (2008). *What is the difference between evaluation and research—and why do we care. Fundamental issues in evaluation*, 183–196.

On Rapid Rural Appraisal
Chambers, R. (2005). *Rural appraisal: Rapid, relaxed, participatory*. Vikas Publishing House.

On Mixed Methods Designs
Greene, J. C., Caracelli, V. J., & Graham, W. F. (1989). *Toward a conceptual framework for mixed-method evaluation designs. Educational evaluation and policy analysis*, 11(3), 255–274. Retrieved from http://citeseerx.ist.psu.edu/viewdoc/ download?doi=10.1.1.456.909&rep=rep1&type=pdf

Chapter questions

1. Define the following terms: evaluation model, evaluation approach, and evaluation design.
2. Describe a rural program or intervention where an evaluation model would be most useful.
3. What is a logic model? How is it used in the evaluation process?
4. List the basic components of a logic model and define these component terms.
5. In your own words, describe the differences between research and evaluation.
6. What are the most common evaluation designs used in rural contexts? What are the strengths and limitations of these designs?
7. What is the difference between research and evaluation?

Practice

1. Review theory-driven evaluation literature. Develop a conceptual model that uses theory-driven evaluation based on a program process theory and a program impact theory.
2. You were just hired by a rural community school to evaluate their teacher training program. This program was just funded and you are planning your first visit to the community. You have been asked to present different evaluation designs, models, and approaches that might be used in the evaluation. How will you prepare for the meeting? What will you bring?
3. Identify a published evaluation article or report from a rural community in the United States. What evaluation approach was used? Is this clearly evaluation or is it research? Did they include a logic model?

References

American Evaluation Association (2014). *What is evaluation?* Retrieved from http://www.eval.org/p/bl/et/blogid=2&blogaid=4

Barley, Z. A., & Jenness, M. (1993). Cluster evaluation: A method to strengthen evaluation in smaller programs with similar purposes. *Evaluation Practice, 14*(2), 141–147.

Bickman, L. (1987). *The functions of program theory using program theory in evaluation. New directions for program evaluation* (Vol. 33). San Francisco, CA: Jossey-Bass.

Blome, J. (2009). *Measuring value. Office of program analysis and evaluation.* National Institute of General Medical Sciences. Retrieved from https://publications.nigms.nih.gov/presentations/measuring_value/index.html

Brinkerhoff, R. O. (2005). The success case method: A strategic evaluation approach to increasing the value and effect of training. *Advances in Developing Human Resources, 7*(1), 86–101.

Bureau of Justice Assistance Center (2011). *Is this a good quality outcome evaluation report? A guide for practitioners.* BJA Center for Program Evaluation and Performance Measurement. Retrieved from https://www.bja.gov/evaluation/reference/Quality_Outcome_Eval.pdf

Centers for Disease Control (1995). *Assessing the effectiveness of disease and injury prevention programs: Costs and consequences. MMRW* August 18, 1995 (RR10); 1–10. Retrieved from https://www.cdc.gov/mmwr/preview/mmwrhtml/00038592.htm

Chambers, R. (1994). The origins and practice of participatory rural appraisal. *World Development, 22*(7), 953–969.

Chambers, R. (2005). Rural appraisal: Rapid, relaxed, participatory In A. Mukherjee (Ed.), *Participatory Rural Appraisal: Methods and Applications in Rural Planning: Essays in Honour of Robert Chambers.* New Delhi: Vikas Publishing House.

Cousins, J. B., & Earl, L. M. (1995). The case for participatory evaluation: Theory, research, practice In L. Cousins & L Earl (Eds.), *Participatory evaluation in education: Studies in evaluation use and organizational learning* (pp. 3–18). Washington, DC: Taylor and Francis Group.

Creswell, J. W. (2013). *Steps in conducting a scholarly mixed methods study.* University of Nebraska Lincoln Presentation. November 14, 2013. Retrieved from: https://digitalcommons. unl.edu/dberspeakers/48/

Donaldson, S. I. (2007). *Program theory-driven evaluation science: Strategies and applications.* New York, NY: Psychology Press.

Drummond, M. F., & McGuire, A. (2001). *Economic evaluation in health care: Merging theory with practice.* Oxford: Oxford University Press.

Dunet, D. (2012). *Centers for disease control and prevention coffee break: Introduction to economic evaluation.* January 10, 2012. Retrieved from https://www.cdc.gov/dhdsp/pubs/docs/ cb_january_10_2012.pdf

Fetterman, D. M. (2001). *Foundations of empowerment evaluation.* Thousand Oaks, CA: Sage Publications.

Fox-Rushby, J. A., & Cairns, J. (2005). *Economic evaluation. Section 1: The structure of economic evaluation.* Maidenhead, NY: Open University Press.

Gertler, P. J., Martinez, S., Premand, P., Rawlings, L. B., & Vermeersch, C. M. J. (2016). *Impact evaluation in practice,* 2nd edition. World Bank Publications. Retrieved from https://ebookcentral-proquest-com.libproxy.uncg.edu

Greene, J. C., Caracelli, V. J., & Graham, W. F. (1989). Toward a conceptual framework for mixed-method evaluation designs. *Educational Evaluation and Policy Analysis, 11*(3), 255–274.

Grosse, S. D., Teutsch, S. M., & Haddix, A. C. (2007). Lessons from cost-effectiveness research for United States public health policy. *Annual Review of Public Health, 28,* 365–391.

Hearn, S (2015). *Developing a theory of change with outcome mapping. Outcome mapping practitioner guide.* Retrieved from https://www.outcomemapping.ca/nuggets/developing-a-theory-of-change-with-outcome-mapping

Hogan, R. L. (2007). The historical development of program evaluation: Exploring past and present. *Online Journal for Workforce Education and Development, 2*(4), 5.

Kaplan, S. A., & Garrett, K. E. (2005). The use of logic models by community-based initiatives. *Evaluation and Program Planning, 28*(2), 167–172.

Khandker, S. R., Koolwal, G. B., & Samad, H. A. (2010). *Handbook on impact evaluation: Quantitative methods and practices.* Washington, DC: World Bank.

Kirkpatrick, D. (1996). Revisiting Kirkpatrick's four-level model. *Training and Development, 50*(1), 54–59.

Mathison, S. (2008). What is the difference between evaluation and research—And why do we care. In N. L. Smith & P. R. Brandon (Eds.), *Fundamental issues in evaluation* (pp. 183–196). New York, NY: Guilford Press.

McLaughlin, J. A., & Jordan, G. B. (1999). Logic models: A tool for telling your programs performance story. *Evaluation and Program Planning, 22*(1), 65–72.

Merriam-Webster (ND). *Research definition.* Retrieved from https://www.merriam-webster.com/dictionary/research

Monette, D., Sullivan, T., & DeJong, C. (1990). *Applied social research: A tool for human services,* 2nd edition. Dallas Fort Worth, TX: Holt, Rinehard, and Winston. p. 337

Newcomer, K. E., Hatry, H. P., & Wholey, J. S. (1994). *Meeting the need for practical evaluation approaches: An introduction. Handbook of practical program evaluation.* San Francisco, CA: Jossey-Bass Inc.

Office for Victims of Crime (2010). *Guide to Performance Measurement and Program Evaluation.* Retrieved from: https://www.ovcttac.gov/docs/resources/OVCTAGuides/PerformanceMeasurement/whatarepm_pfv.html

Organization for Economic Co-operation and Development (2018). *DAC Criteria for Evaluating Development Assistance.* Retrieved from http://www.oecd.org/dac/evaluation/daccriteriaforevaluatingdevelopmentassistance.htm

Owen, J. M. (2007). *Program evaluation: Forms and approaches.* New York, NY: Guilford Press. doi:10.4135/9781849209601.n12

Patton, M. Q. (2008). *Utilization-focused evaluation.* Thousand Oaks, CA: Sage Publications.

Phelps, C., & Mushlin, A. (1991) On the near equivalence of cost-effectiveness and cost-benefit analyses. *International Journal of Technology Assessment in Health Care, 7,* 12–21.

Preskill, H., & Russ-Eft, D. (2004). *Building evaluation capacity: 72 activities for teaching and training.* Thousand Oaks, CA: Sage Publications.

Robinson, R. (1993). Cost-benefit analysis. *BMJ, 307,* 859–862.

Saunders, R. P., Evans, M. H., & Joshi, P. (2005). Developing a process-evaluation plan for assessing health promotion program implementation: A how-to guide. *Health Promotion Practice, 6*(2), 134–147. doi:10.1177/1524839904273387

Savaya, R., & Waysman, M. (2005). The logic model: A tool for incorporating theory in development and evaluation of programs. *Administration in Social Work, 29*(2), 85–103.

Scheirer, M. A. (1994). Designing and using process evaluation. In J. S Wholey, H. P. Hatry & K. E. Newcomer (Eds.), *Handbook of practical program evaluation,* Ch. 3. San Francisco, CA: Jossey-Bass.

Stufflebeam, D. L. (1985). Stufflebeam's improvement-oriented evaluation. In D. L. Stufflebeam & A. J. Shinkfield (Eds.), *Systematic evaluation* (pp. 151–207). Dordrecht: Springer.

Stufflebeam, D. L., Madaus, G. F., & Kellaghan, T. (Eds.). (2000). *Evaluation models: Viewpoints on educational and human services evaluation* (Vol. 49). New York, NY: Springer Science & Business Media.

Substance Abuse and Mental Health Services Administration (2017). *Cooperative agreements to implement zero suicide in health systems.* FOA No. SM 17-006, CFDA No. 93.243. Retrieved from: https://www.samhsa.gov/grants/grant-announcements/sm-17-006

Tennant, C., Boonkrong, M., & Roberts, P. A. (2002). The design of a training programme measurement model. *Journal of European Industrial Training, 26*(5), 230–240.

Wandersman, A., Keener, D. C., Snell-Johns, J., Miller, R. L., Flaspohler, P., Livet-Dye, M., et al. (2004). Empowerment evaluation: Principles and action. In L. A. Jason, C. B. Keys, Y. Suarez-Balcazar, R. R. Taylor, & M. I. Davis (Eds.), *Participatory community research: Theories and methods in action* (pp. 139–156). Washington, DC: American Psychological Association.

Warr, P., Bird, M., & Rackham, N. (1970). *Evaluation of management training: A practical framework, with cases, for evaluating training needs and results.* London: Gower Press.

Wholey, J. S. (2004). Evaluability assessment. In J. S Wholey, H. P. Hatry, K. E. Newcomer (Eds.), *Handbook of practical program evaluation* (pp. 33–62). 2nd edition. San Francisco, CA: Jossey-Bass.

Williams, B. L., & Suen, H. K. (1998). Formal versus informal assessment methods. *American Journal of Health Behavior, 22*(4), 308–313.

Zechmeister, E. B., Shaughnessy, J. J., & Zechmeister, J. S. (1996). *A practical introduction to research methods in psychology.* New York, NY: McGraw-Hill Humanities Social.

5

THE RURAL COMMUNITY EVALUATION PROCESS

I can do things you cannot, you can do things I cannot; together we can do great things.

—Mother Teresa

What I wish I would have known when I started my career as an evaluator working in rural communities...I wish someone would have told me that there are many ways to do rural evaluation, there is not a one-size-fits-all approach. I also think the time in the community is something that has made me more effective, and taking time to be in a community, to get to know people, and allow them to know me is worth more than any report or measure. There are so many things that happen in a rural evaluation that are not documented in the rural evaluation planning process. It is hard, for example, to quantify the strength of relationships, the trust that is established within programs, and the time that it takes.

Planning

Planning for program evaluation in rural communities may occur before a program is implemented, during implementation, or in some cases, after a program has occurred. Ideally, planning the evaluation occurs at the beginning of the program in conjunction with initial program planning efforts. But, in rural communities, funding is often limited and evaluators may not be hired until after a program has been designed and implementation begins (Figure 5.1).

Regardless of when the rural evaluation planning process begins, these guidelines will help programs as they plan for evaluation:

1. Engage with stakeholders and determine what questions they want answered in the evaluation.
2. Know the program goals and objectives that you are evaluating.

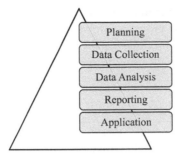

FIGURE 5.1 Five Basic Elements of Rural Evaluation.

3. Identify resources available for the evaluation, the overall budget, and program costs.
4. Hire an evaluator.
5. Design the evaluation.
6. Select evaluation instruments that will be used in the evaluation.
7. Make sure that the evaluation questions address the goals and objectives of the program.
8. Ensure that questions from all stakeholder groups are considered in the evaluation.
9. Develop a time line for the evaluation.

Engaging stakeholders and community members

When we think about engaging stakeholders and community in rural evaluation, we must acknowledge and know their unique history. For example, When was the community established? By Whom? Who were the original inhabitants? How did the community get its name? Who are the people that live in the community? What are they known for? What have they overcome? What is the pace of life in the community? Answering these questions will help, as we consider ways to engage stakeholders in the rural evaluation process.

Engaging stakeholders is first step in the rural community evaluation process. To begin, stakeholders are the people or organizations that are involved in a program that have an interest (or stake) in the evaluation. In rural communities, stakeholders may include churches, first responders, teachers, schools, hospitals, clinics, city council men and women, community members, volunteers, elders, business owners, farmers, nonprofit organizations, and others. Stakeholders can also be funders, grant makers, and evaluators/researchers. The term engagement refers to the process of bringing people (stakeholders and community) together for the purpose of a common goal. Previous authors established the importance of community engagement and the benefits of community engaged evaluation (Ahmed & Palermo, 2010). When communities are involved in the evaluation process, the outcomes are more meaningful, the interventions are more appropriate, and the program efforts are more likely to be sustained. But what does it really mean to engage stakeholders and community members in rural evaluation? This is a meaningful question before beginning work with a community.

Building trust

Evaluators are often outsiders, they may be affiliated with a university, a state, or local government, or they might be independent consultants (Wallerstein, 1999). Rural evaluators must establish trust with the communities they are working with early in the evaluation process. Effective communication is critical for trust building. Evaluators must plan for communication before, throughout, and during the evaluation process. Communication supports the trust building process by ensuring that the rural evaluation process is clear and the intentions of the evaluator are known. Evaluators can also build trust by sharing information widely. When people feel they are left out of the conversation, or they are not receiving all of the information, this creates distrust and a feeling of disrespect. It is best to allow all stakeholders to provide feedback on an issue, and it is likely that there are different perspectives on a certain issue (Figure 5.2).

Respect

Respect is critical in building trust. Respect must be genuine and authentic. When evaluators do not respect community and stakeholders, they will not be respected either. As evaluators, we can demonstrate respect by treating others with kindness, being polite, encouraging community members to share their ideas, and then using these ideas in the evaluation process. Being transparent is also critical for rural evaluators. Evaluators' should not have hidden agendas and must be honest about their role and the role of community and stakeholders in the evaluation process. Sharing information with community members will create an environment of trust and value in the community. Last, evaluators can earn the trust and respect in communities by providing concrete ways for communities to

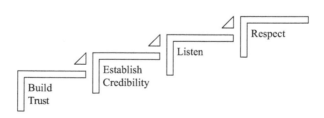

FIGURE 5.2 Steps for Engaging Stakeholders.

engage in the evaluation process (Jagosh et al., 2015). The pathways to building trust and respect in rural community evaluation occur over time. Considerations for building trust and respect in rural evaluation include engaging stakeholders, getting acquainted, establishing a framework for trust, experiencing and resolving conflict, and time. The literature on Community-Based Participatory Research does a good job of operationalizing trust and respect for evaluators and rural communities (Minkler, 2004). What trust looks like in the evaluation process may vary by rural community, evaluator, and context—these elements are a good place to start.

Establish credibility

In the evaluation process, there are two different kinds of credibility that may be discussed. The first type of credibility in evaluation refers to the kinds of evidence used in evaluation—Mertens and Hesse-Biber wrote an entire book on the topic, *Mixed Methods and Credibility of Evidence in Evaluation* (2013). Credibility of evidence used in rural evaluation is extremely important, but I want you to consider the concept of establishing your credibility as an evaluator. Have you ever met someone and thought that they might not be credible? This might have been a doctor, a teacher, a speaker, or even a preacher. What was it about them that made you question their credibility? Alternately, have you met someone that you immediately trusted? What was it about them that made you feel this way?

As a rural community evaluator, your credibility is important. First, let people know who you are. Without the titles, degrees, job affiliations, or status, demonstrate who you are by your actions rather than words. Be honest early in the evaluation process, letting people know your strengths and weaknesses is a sure way to build your credibility and their trust. Also, spend time in the community and get proximate to what is happening. Finally, have examples available of rural evaluations that you have completed. Provide references, resources, and guidance documents that show your level of knowledge and expertise in rural evaluation (Box 5.1).

BOX 5.1 Field notes on trust and credibility

I let rural communities know that my strengths are managing large data sets, thinking about the big picture, and technical writing. I tell people that, as an evaluator, I can get sidetracked with good ideas and conversations. Sometimes I lack attention to detail that is needed to conduct rural evaluation. I am not perfect.

TABLE 5.1 Active Listening Strategies

LADDERS to Active Listening

Look at the person you are talking with if it is appropriate for the community and
  culture you are working with. Use body language to let them know you are listening.
Ask questions. Make comments when the speaker is finished talking.
Don't interrupt.
Don't change the subject.
Emotions should be neutral. Identify with the speaker's emotions when possible. Find
  common ground.
Respond appropriately based on context and culture.
Slow down. Quiet your mind and really think about the speaker's message.

Source: Adapted from Jalongo (2008), Learning to listen, listening to learn. *Washington, DC: National Association for the Education of Young Children.*

Listen

Listening is essential for engaging rural communities and stakeholders in the evaluation process. Cultural differences should be accounted for when considering active listening strategies. For example, in some rural and Native communities, it is not polite to look at the person you are talking with. Table 5.1 outlines active listening strategies.

The perspectives and ideas that stakeholders share are invaluable in the evaluation process. Their ideas will help shape a useful evaluation by helping frame key evaluation questions, supporting work plan development, and ensuring that evaluation findings reflect stakeholder views and priorities. Can you imagine an evaluation plan that did not include the voices and perspectives of stakeholders? By practicing active listening, asking questions, don't interrupt, don't change subject, emotions are neutral, respond appropriately (LADDER) technique (Jalongo, 2008), evaluators can be sure that the voice, message, and ideas are implemented into the evaluation plan. Now that we have covered the basic elements of engaging stakeholders, let us consider how to support communities as they develop program goals and objectives.

Goals and objectives in the evaluation plan

A **goal** is what the community hopes to achieve as a result of the program. Goals should be developed in partnership with community. Consider the following questions:

- What is the vision of the rural organization/community?
- What is their mission?
- What is the problem statement or focus area of the evaluation?
- How does the goal address the problem statement?

How do evaluators develop evaluation goals with community participation?

Develop goals using a participatory process. The literature on Empowerment Evaluation techniques highlights how evaluators can facilitate the process of goal development in the evaluation planning process (Fetterman & Wandersman, 2007).

In recent years, there has been a shift in how funding agencies want goals written. For example, some want Specific Measurable Achievable Relevant and Time-bound (SMART) goals (see Figure 5.3), and others want broad visionary goals supported by measurable objectives (Rubin, 2002). Either way, the best way to write and implement goals and objectives is with community input and following funding agency guidelines (Figure 5.3).

Objectives

Once you have established your program goals, you will need to develop objectives that describe the results that you hope to achieve and how they will be achieved. Using the same SMART framework, objectives can be process or outcome oriented.

Objectives should be clearly defined, observable, measurable, and valid. Possible questions that can help when designing objectives include the following:

- What are we going to do?
- What is it important for us to accomplish this activity?

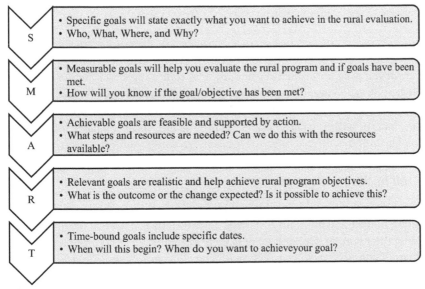

S
- Specific goals will state exactly what you want to achieve in the rural evaluation.
- Who, What, Where, and Why?

M
- Measurable goals will help you evaluate the rural program and if goals have been met.
- How will you know if the goal/objective has been met?

A
- Achievable goals are feasible and supported by action.
- What steps and resources are needed? Can we do this with the resources available?

R
- Relevant goals are realistic and help achieve rural program objectives.
- What is the outcome or the change expected? Is it possible to achieve this?

T
- Time-bound goals include specific dates.
- When will this begin? When do you want to achieveyour goal?

Source: Adapted from Rubin (2002).

FIGURE 5.3 Developing SMART Goals and Objectives.

- Who is going to be responsible for the activities?
- When do we want this to be completed?
- How are we going to do these activities?

We will use these concepts later in this chapter when we discuss work plans and designing the rural evaluation plan.

Identify resources available

Resources available for the evaluation may include community assets, the evaluation budget, and program costs.

Rural communities may have different resources available for evaluation. Examples include the United States Department of Agriculture (USDA), Extension offices, state grants that are administered through county offices, community colleges, community groups, and others. Generally, there are fewer resources available for program implementation and evaluation in rural communities. When thinking about the evaluation process, it is important to work with the community to develop a list of community resources or assets. Sometimes this process is called asset mapping (see Figure 5.4). What are some differences in rural community assets compared with urban community assets? What about the distance it takes to access these resources? Figure 5.4 lists resources available in city and urban locations that are 30–130 miles away.

Knowing community resources and assets will help develop a realistic evaluation and program budget. In many cases, evaluators and programs leverage existing resources in the community to support the evaluation. This is particularly important when funding agencies require a budget match.

Evaluation budgets

When developing an evaluation budget, the following cost categories are included: staffing, materials and supplies, equipment, and travel. Consider who will be conducting the evaluation, what the evaluation will include, and where the evaluation will take place. If you are feeling like you need more information on budgeting, don't panic, we will learn more about budgeting in Chapter 9.

Overall budget and program costs

Another resource available for the evaluation is the program budget. The overall program budget and program costs will be driven by the agency or organization funding the program. Because there is such variability in rural program budgets, evaluators will need to work closely with the community, stakeholders, and program staff to understand the budget requirements and costs for implementing the program goals and objectives (Box 5.2).

Educational Support
Materials and supplies for low income families
Parenting Classes
Schools

Mental Health
Youth and Family Services Counseling
Youth Counseling-C
Behavioral Health
Dept. Health & Human Services Psychiatric
Hospitalization-U

Churches
Catholic Church x 2
Baptist
Catholic Church
Latter Day Saints
Non-Denominational

Substance Abuse Help
Drug and Alcohol Prevention
Recovery Center for Treatment
Behavioral Health for Counseling
Youth Counseling-C
Access to Recovery for Treatment-U
In Patient Chemical Dependency Center <18 years-U
Church-Based 12 Step Program

Food
WIC, SNAP for Low Income
Commodity Food Program

Shelter & Housing Support
Lodge Shelter for Children
Housing Authority,
Housing Assistance Council
Family Services-Child Residential
Care and Clothing
Youth Dynamics for Emergency Shelter
Runaway Program-U

Recreation & Activities
Boys and Girls Clubs
Youth Groups

Juvenile Justice
Courts
Law Enforcement
Juvenile Probation Officer

Medical Services
Clinic
City Memorial Hospital-C
Urban Hospital-U

Abuse
Social Services
Child Family Services-U

*C=City Location 30 miles, U-Urban Location 120 miles

FIGURE 5.4 Field Notes on Rural Community Asset Map for Substance Abuse and Mental Health Services Administration (SAMHSA) Grant.

BOX 5.2 Field notes on evaluation budgets

As an independent evaluator, I work with communities based on the funds they have available for the evaluation. I typically charge an hourly rate and often subcontract with other evaluators to support data collection or on-the-ground efforts in communities. If a community has $40,000 a year for a program evaluation, I will consider their priorities, what will be the best use of their funds, and how to leverage community resources to support a comprehensive and meaningful evaluation.

TABLE 5.2 Budget Guidelines Example

USDA Office of Community Food Systems Rural Planning Grant Guidelines	
Funding range	$20,000–$50,000
Time line	12 or 24 months
Food costs	No more than 10% of the budget can be used for food
Match	A 25% match is required
Unallowable costs	Equipment is not an allowable expense
Evaluation	Not included in the guidelines, generally no more than 20% of total budget

Source: United States Department of Agriculture (2018).

Most grants have a funding range, time line, and budget restraints. Table 5.2 provides an example from the USDA 2018 Farm to School Grant Program.

Community concerns: the needs of the community

Rural evaluators must know the concerns of the community. This is often accomplished early in the proposal writing process, where funding agencies require documentation of need to fund a given problem. Sometimes this process is called a needs assessment. The Rural Health Information Hub has an excellent resource for conducting a needs assessment in rural communities (https://www.rural-healthinfo.org/community-health/rural-toolkit/1/needs-assessment). Depending on where you are at in the evaluation process, it might be useful to examine concerns based on potential risks or threats to the program being implemented. Table 5.3 is an example of how evaluators can work with rural communities to identify needs in the evaluation process.

TABLE 5.3 Field Notes on Identifying Community Concerns in Practice

Community Concerns from a Rural Suicide Prevention Program	
Limited resources to support prevention and treatment.	Crisis nature in the community makes it difficult to plan and fully engage community and leaders. "It is only an issue or important after it has happened".
Program does not work closely with clinical program to share referral information.	Difficulty in documenting the impact of prevention program due to small numbers, emerging data capacity and resources.
Burnout of staff to carryout project goals and objectives.	Changes in staffing and limited prevention workforce.
Rural and isolated community—long distances between districts and external resources necessary for treatment.	Lack of consistency between programs and services create challenges for implementing consistent prevention messaging and outreach.

Work plan

A **work plan** is a way of tracking project goals, objectives, resources, and due dates. Work plans may be required by funding agencies and submitted with quarterly or semiannual reports. They may also be used internally to make sure a program is on track to meet its goals and objectives (Table 5.4).

After you draft your work plan, it will be necessary to develop measurable outcomes. Table 5.5 provides an example; keep in mind that you will have several objectives and outcomes in your work plan.

TABLE 5.4 Field Notes on Goals and Tracking

Goal 1: Strengthen the Coping Skills of 150 High School Youth

Objectives (What, How Many?)	Activities to Achieve Objective	Person Responsible (Who?)	Date Due	Resources Required (Funding, Facilities, staff)	Comments
Develop, pilot, and evaluate a 40-hour life skills curriculum for 150 9th–12th graders at Riverton High School.	1 Finalize and pilot curriculum at one location. 2 Meet with schools and develop schedule for implementation 3 Offer curriculum throughout the year. 4 Administer pre/post COPE Scale	Jane Smith	August 31, 2018	$10,500 supplies Local High School Class Room 100 hours/ staff time Jane Smith	Memorandum of Understanding (MOU) OU in place for curriculum. Funding for supplies must be approved prior to 10/17

TABLE 5.5 Field Notes on Outcome Measures in Work Plan

Measurable Outcomes Goal 1: Strengthen the Coping Skills of 150 High School Youth

Outcome Measure (How Objective Was Measured)	Date Accomplished	Results	Resources Used	Comments
Sign-in sheets from high school classes	June 15, 2018	161 students	$8,777 contracts $2,300 and travel funds 90-hour staff time Interventionist	Seven classes implemented from December 2017–June 2018 MOU was helpful in supporting facility use and data collection.
Increased scores for COPE scale items based on pre/post data.	June 15, 2018	Mean increase of 4.5, $p < 0.01$	COPE scale-14 items	Overall mean increases in pre/post mean scores demonstrate impact.

BOX 5.3 Field notes on work plans

I was working as the lead evaluator in rural Montana. I worked with the community to write a work plan that would meet the grant requirements and deadlines—the only problem with the work plan we developed was it was not realistic. The funding agency required staff to be hired within the first 30 days of the grant award, but the community human resource policy required that a staff position be posted for 30 days before interviews took place. We spoke with our project officer and received an extension to meet the grant requirements.

Evaluators in rural communities are often tasked with developing a work plan for a program that is then used to develop the evaluation plan. You might be wondering, "What is the difference between a work plan and an evaluation plan?" Work plans are written documents that can be used by program staff to track action steps/objectives, person responsible, due dates, and activities. Evaluation plans are often used to develop the work plan, but they are different. An evaluation plan outlines the planning, data collection strategy, data analysis plan, reporting, and application of results (see Figure 5.1).

It may be necessary to create two work plans, one with the funding agency requirements and the other for the community to review. By working with stakeholders and the community, evaluators can develop and refine a work plan based on changing resources, staffing, and context—flexibility in developing and following a work plan is often needed. Work plans are useful when they are developed with the community and provide clear and concise guidance that aligns with the funding agency requirements and program plans. In other instances, work plans are not as useful (Box 5.3).

Finally, the language that we use when developing evaluation work plans must match community definitions. For example, using the term action step rather than objective may be more meaningful to rural communities. Now that we have an understanding of work plans, let's learn more about designing a rural evaluation plan.

Designing the evaluation plan

First, let's consider some basic questions about evaluation plans using the probes of What, How, Who, When, and Why.

> *What?* An evaluation plan is a written document that outlines the plan for evaluating a program.
>
> *How?* Four main steps guide the evaluation planning process. First, clarify the program objectives and goals. Second, develop evaluation questions.

Third, develop evaluation methods that are appropriate for the rural community. Fourth, create a timeline for evaluation activities.

Who? The evaluation plan is typically created by the evaluator with the input from the stakeholders and community.

When? Evaluation plans are first outlined in a proposal, then revised after a program is funded but before a program begins. This process varies based on the reasons for the evaluation and funding agency requirements.

Why? Evaluation plans help us know what is working what is not. Evaluation plans also help us identify a process for assessing barriers and challenges along with the necessary resources for implementing a program. Evaluation plans can help determine the impact of a given program and the results related to cost savings, reach of activities, and overall outcomes.

In practice, evaluation plans are critical. It is important to keep in mind that evaluation plans can change based on what is happening in a community or program (Box 5.4).

A solid evaluation design is crucial for rural evaluation. Here are some recommendations on what the evaluation design should include:

Summary information about the program
Questions that will be addressed by the evaluation
Data collection strategies that will be used
People/groups who will implement activities
When the activities will be conducted
Products of the evaluation including who will receive them and how they should be used.
Projected costs to do the evaluation.

BOX 5.4 Field notes on designing an evaluation plan

Several years ago, I was the lead evaluator on a grant for a small nonprofit in a rural community. The goal of the grant was to determine gaps in the system of care for children and families with severe mental health needs. About a year into the program, the nonprofit and community determined that the funding agency definition of a system of care did not match the community definition of a system of care. This required a major change in the evaluation plan, goals, and objectives. Language is important and while there are different ways that we can define elements in the evaluation, it is critical that rural evaluators know community definitions and terms used in the evaluation process.

In Chapter 4, we learned about evaluation designs, approaches, and models. You might recall that evaluation designs are typically viewed as experimental, quasi-experimental, nonexperimental, or mixed methods. Most rural program evaluations fall into the mixed methods, nonexperimental or quasi-experimental design categories. Many rural evaluations are process, outcome, or impact focused. Conceptual frameworks and theories are also used when designing the evaluation plan. The next section summarizes these important tools for rural evaluation purposes.

Conceptual framework

The **conceptual framework** organizes ideas and concepts about a particular program or intervention with attention to the program's data and goals. Conceptual frameworks are often part or all of the logic model because the model includes inputs, outputs, and outcomes. Conceptual frameworks are necessary in rural evaluation because they outline how a program is expected to work to achieve desired goals. Most evaluators will develop a conceptual framework based on a theory. Figure 5.4 is a conceptual framework from a rural intervention project.

Theories

Theories are ideas about what will happen given an intervention or program. Generally grounded in literature and science, some theories may not be a good fit for the rural community or program being evaluated. If you are having a difficult time selecting a theory for the evaluation, talk with a colleague, or read literature on theory-driven evaluation (Fitzpatrick, Sanders, & Wortehn, 2004; Lipsey & Pollard, 1989; Patton, 2008). Reviewing the kinds of theories that are being used in the field or discipline may be useful when selecting a theory (Rogers, 2014). Funding agencies may also have resources available (Box 5.5).

Theories are useful because they can help evaluators describe what they think will happen as a result of a program based on a program strategy (Bickman, 1987). The if–then thinking described in Figure 5.5 is an example of how the theory of change can be applied to rural evaluation programs.

BOX 5.5 Field notes on theories

One theory that I have used numerous times as a rural evaluator is the theory of change. Evaluators may use a theory of change to understand more about the results that come from a program. The theory of change is most appropriate when objectives and activities are identified and planned with a community. Ideally, this occurs before the program begins and prompts ideas and discussion about what will change as a result of a program (Rogers, 2014).

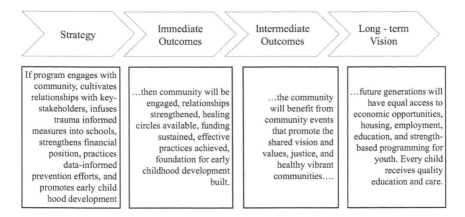

Strategy	Immediate Outcomes	Intermediate Outcomes	Long - term Vision
If program engages with community, cultivates relationships with key-stakeholders, infuses trauma informed measures into schools, strengthens financial position, practices data-informed prevention efforts, and promotes early child hood development	...then community will be engaged, relationships strengthened, healing circles available, funding sustained, effective practices achieved, foundation for early childhood development built.	...the community will benefit from community events that promote the shared vision and values, justice, and healthy vibrant communities....	...future generations will have equal access to economic opportunities, housing, employment, education, and strength-based programming for youth. Every child receives quality education and care.

FIGURE 5.5   Field Notes on a Rural Program Theory of Change.

Time lines

There are two time lines that evaluators must consider in the evaluation plan: the first is the overall program time line. This includes major milestones, due dates, reporting requirements, and individuals responsible. The work plan may be useful in developing a program time line. The second time line supports data collection. In this section, we will focus on time lines to support data collection. There are three different times that data is usually collected, before the program begins, during the program, and after it has been completed. When data is collected depends on the goals and objectives of the evaluation and the evaluation design. For example, if you are measuring the impact of a life skills intervention, you may want to collect baseline data before the intervention begins; this is generally a **pretest/ posttest design**. This type of design can help you determine what skills students had before the intervention and changes that resulted from the intervention. You may also need to collect data during an intervention to determine if changes are needed, this is often called a time-series design. Consider a **time–series design** for observing changes over time using select indicators at multiple time points. Time-series designs are experimental designs that involve one group of people who are exposed to a program or intervention (Fraenkel, Wallen, & Hyun, 1993). Data is collected repeatedly before the program (pretested) and after the program (posttested). Finally, data can be collected after a program is completed to determine program impacts and lessons learned. This type of design is considered a nonexperimental **posttest-only** design. All designs have strengths and limitations; know these before you begin planning your data collection time line.

Data collection plan

Data collection is perhaps the most essential aspect of the evaluation plan. In Chapter 6, we will learn more about data collection and analysis—in this chapter, we focus on the elements of data collection that should be included in the rural evaluation plan.

Data collection strategy

Rural evaluators can work with communities to develop a data collection strategy. This should be highlighted in the evaluation plan and include the following information:

> Define population of interest—define the group or unit, the geographical area of interests, and the time/year(s) of interest.
> Summarize the sampling (collection) strategy—probability, purposive, or convenience.
> Consider the kinds of data that will be collected and the reliability and validity of these data.
> Determine how data collected relates to the goals and objectives of the program.
> Develop plan for addressing dropouts and refusals.
> Identify how the data will be collected, entered, analyzed, and shared.
> Practice sound data management.

Examples of data that may be collected in rural communities are outlined in Table 5.6.

TABLE 5.6 Field Notes on Data in Rural Evaluation

Data Source	Data Type	Data Purpose	Collection Strategy[a]
Surveys	Qualitative, quantitative, or both	Document ideas, perceptions, feedback	In-person, mail, telephone, or online
Pre- and posttests	Quantitative	Document changes based on program participation	In-person or online
Focus groups	Qualitative	Collect feedback from groups about program	In-person
Interviews	Qualitative	Collect information about program and impacts	In-person
Photographs, art, videos, drawings, or images	Qualitative	Document context, visual depictions, can be used to assess program changes (i.e. before and after photo)	In-person
Program documentation	Qualitative, quantitative, or both	Document outputs, outcomes, and impacts of program	Existing data from reports, materials, sign-in sheets, administrative data, and other sources

a Some evaluators facilitate focus groups and interviews using web-based technology, online meeting spaces, and other audio video technology. Before deciding on a data collection strategy in a rural community, consult with stakeholders to determine norms, preferences, and preferred communication strategies.

Data ownership

After you know the kinds of data you will be collecting, work with the community to determine who has legal rights to the data and who retains the data after the project ends. In some cases, the funding agency has specific requirements about data ownership and how the data will be treated and disseminated. Because data ownership varies by funding agency, community, and program, this should be outlined early in the evaluation planning process.

Data agreements

Determine early on how data will be used in the evaluation. Data use agreements may be necessary when using administrative data for evaluation purposes; in some cases, these data are confidential and require evaluators to sign an agreement agreeing to certain terms and conditions. Data use agreements are essential for evaluators because they include limitation on the use of data, safeguarding the data, liability from harm from use of data, publication, and privacy rights.

Data management

Evaluation results in data that is generated as a result of the program. Good data management requires evaluators to consistently collect and record data, store data securely, clean data, transfer data, present data, and make data accessible to other users when appropriate. The type of data storage that you need depends on the kind of data that you have. When you are developing consent forms for the evaluation, make sure you include information about how the data will be used and stored. It is also important to consider the types of storage options available, for example, select data storage based on electronic vs. paper files, access to a secure file location, and the number of years the data will need to be stored.

Who collects data?

Data may be collected by the evaluator, community members, youth, interns, volunteers, partners, or program staff. When considering who will collect evaluation data, consider the history of the community, the norms, and the use of trusted individuals. Some communities distrust outsiders, if you are an evaluator from the outside—it may be difficult to collect data. In such cases, I encourage evaluators to work with program staff and trusted community members to collect data. Evaluators can train these individuals and support the data collection process without being the person that collects the data.

Small sample size

One of the unique challenges of working in rural communities is the small population. It is important for evaluators to determine the number of people that live in the community, the number of people in the target population based on age and gender (when appropriate). Using the evaluation design process mentioned earlier in this chapter, evaluators will want to select an evaluation design that is appropriate for the size of the population. Previous authors have said that there is no standard sample size. Sample size is dependent on the evaluation questions, what the community hopes the evaluation will achieve, and the resources available. If you are collecting quantitative data, statistical formulas will give you the sample size needed. If you are collecting qualitative data, it is recommended that the sample is representative of the community or the target population served by the program.

Measuring results of program with best data available

Primary data is data that is collected by the program or evaluator. An example of primary data is a survey that is developed with the community to determine resources and concerns regarding substance use. In contrast, **secondary data**, or sometimes called **administrative data**, is collected by someone else, but is available to the evaluator. Examples of secondary data include intake forms, attendance rosters, program logs, evaluation forms, case files, follow-up data, and assessments. Other **extant data** includes census data, vital statistics data, crime statistics, national survey data, and community profile data. An example of an extant data source is the United States Department of Agriculture Economic Research Service database (https://www.ers.usda.gov/data-products.aspx). This data set could be used to analyze the impact of education on persistent child poverty by county.

When considering how you will measure the results of a program using primary, secondary, or extant data, it is important to consider the advantages and disadvantages of each. Primary data is specific to the problem being investigated, the data quality can be better, and if the community determines that additional data is needed, it can be collected. Administrative data has already been collected, so the time and funding required to collect the data is minimal; however, administrative data may not match the program or intervention goals, target population, or time line. Regardless of the data source, keep in mind that when evaluating rural programs, it is necessary to be innovative using the best available data for the population and evaluation questions (Box 5.6).

BOX 5.6 Field notes on data collection

In 2013, I was working in a rural North Carolina community with a team to evaluate the effectiveness of a school-based intervention to reduce HIV risk behaviors. We collected primary data from middle school girls. Data included the child's name, date of birth, address, medical history, phone number, and survey responses. These data were handled with extreme care. After surveys were entered into a password-protected database, they were stored in a locked file cabinet in a separate office. All identifying information was removed. Consent forms, photographs, program reports, sign-in sheets, and evaluation forms were stored in a secure location. Rural evaluators have a major responsibility to ensure sound data management practices. This is not always easy, but it is required.

Institutional Review Boards

Evaluation plans should address the Institutional Review Board (IRB) process, time line, and requirements. IRBs were established by congress in 1974 to regulate federally funded research and evaluation studies (US Department of Health and Human Services, ND). The primary role of IRBs is to minimize risks to human subjects. IRBs in rural communities may be located at the hospital or community college, or they may be associated with a funding agency, university, or centralized IRB resource. Evaluators can search for IRBs in the US Department of Health and Human Services Office of Human Research Protections database (https://ohrp. cit.nih.gov/search/SrchMtch.aspx). During the planning process, evaluators need to work closely with the program staff to determine the community protocols for submitting evaluation to IRBs. When working with tribal sovereign nations, evaluators must be aware of how tribes define and approve evaluation/research—this is often different than non-tribal evaluations (Kelley, Belcourt-Dittloff, Belcourt, & Belcourt, 2013). Once the evaluation plan is developed, rural evaluators may submit an IRB application to the appropriate IRB of record. Evaluations are often exempt from IRB review if they do not use identifiable information. For more on IRBs, visit the additional resources section at the end of this chapter.

Performance measures and outcomes

Performance measures

The evaluation plan often includes evaluation performance measures. **Performance measures** track the program accomplishments and progress toward goals. Often performance measures include data on the kinds of activities (inputs) and products or services (outputs) resulting from a program (see Logic Models). Evaluators often work with the funding agency, community, and program staff to define performance measures. Performance measures are beneficial because they tell what a program did and how well it was done.

Outcomes

When you consider outcomes in the evaluation plan, remember that they are the intended initial, intermediate, and final result of an activity. **Outcomes** can be a desired change in behavior, attitude, knowledge, skills, or conditions at the individual, agency, system, or community level. Outcomes are different from outputs (services or activities). Short-term outcomes are typically one to three years, whereas long-term outcomes are three to five years. Outcomes can be difficult to link with a program or intervention being evaluated. This is especially true when there is a small population size, and exposure to multiple programs—this makes it difficult to isolate the program effects and determine if outcomes are actually related to the short- or long-term changes observed. Limited sample sizes and nonsignificant impacts of differences are common challenges that evaluators experience. Sound sampling strategies that match program outcomes are one way to document the short- and long-term outcomes of a given program. There may be unintended outcomes that result from a program or intervention; these can be both positive and negative. Rural evaluators can help community members and stakeholders determine outcomes and how to utilize lessons learned to improve programs if they include outcomes in their evaluation plan.

Plan for sharing results

The evaluation plan should include how evaluation results will be shared and used to improve programs, policies, resources, and effectiveness. Make sure that you include a dissemination plan in your evaluation plan—even if the plan changes, this will help identify the target audience, dissemination mediums to be used, the frequency and date of communications, the person responsible, and any follow-up activities (Table 5.7).

TABLE 5.7 Field Notes on Dissemination Plan

Audience	Dissemination Medium (Print, Electronic, Verbal)	Frequency or Date	Responsible Person	Follow-up Activities
Health program staff	Presentations at site coordinator meetings	Quarterly	Jane	Meeting with staff to clarify questions
Policy makers	Print evaluation brief, verbal presentation	Quarterly	Don	Call to policy makers to determine action taken
Community stakeholders	Print and electronic report in community newsletter	Quarterly	Jane	Review of how many people downloaded electronic report, number of print reports shared
Policy makers and community stakeholders	Article for community newsletter, briefings to community groups	Annually or as appropriate	Sara	Meeting with program staff to discuss briefings and community reaction
Community stakeholders	Community outcomes processes (town hall meetings that reach intended audience)	Annually	Jane, Don, and Sara	Meeting with program staff

Summary

In this chapter, we presented an overview of the rural evaluation planning process. We started with a five-step summary of how to develop a rural evaluation plan: planning, data collection, data analysis, reporting, and application. Engaging stakeholders early in the evaluation process is critical—determine what questions they want answered in the evaluation. There are several ways to engage stakeholders and community; always remember that the process is driven by trust, credibility, and respect. Evaluation plans must include program goals and objectives; these are necessary because they tell us what we are evaluating. SMART goals and objectives are just one of the many ways to develop meaningful and measurable goals and objectives. Designing the evaluation is perhaps the most challenging step in the process. Evaluation designs are not always clear, and often confused because programs require different kinds of designs based on the goal of the program or in some cases intervention. Evaluators must have an understanding of the community, context, history, norms, needs, and resources. Community asset mapping and needs assessments can help inform the evaluation plan. Understanding these critical issues is necessary before beginning to design the evaluation. Evaluation plans can be useful in guiding the evaluation approach, keeping your evaluation on track, and thinking about the big picture of what you are doing and how it will be used in the future. Developing a dissemination plan for the program will help ensure that evaluation results are communicated in a systematic way. In closing, the rural evaluation planning process outlined in this chapter serve as a basic guide. Ultimately this guide is driven by community needs, community resources, and the questions the evaluation seeks to answer.

Points to remember

1 Planning is the first step in designing a rural evaluation.
2. Engaging stakeholders in the planning process is important—determine how they want to be involved and the time that they have available to participate in planning activities.
3. Rural evaluators must work to earn trust and establish credibility in rural communities—especially when they are new to the community or not from a similar background or context.
4. Planning begins with a review of the budget, assessment of community needs and strengths, a work plan, designing the evaluation plan, costs, theories, time line, data collection plan, performance measures, and outcomes.
5. Develop a dissemination plan early in the process. This plan will help you communicate the right information, at the right time, to the intended audience.

Additional reading and resources

On Building Trust
Covey, Stephen (2006). "The Speed of trust: the one thing that changes everything." *Simon and Schuster.*

On Engaging Stakeholders
Better Evaluation (2018). Options. Engage Stakeholders. Retrieved from http://www.betterevaluation.org/en/plan/manage/identify_engage_users

On Evaluation Budgets
Wilder Research (2009). Evaluation on a shoestring budget. Retrieved from http://www.wilder.org/

On Work plans
Health Resources Service Administration Work Plan Example. Retrieved from https://bphc.hrsa.gov/programopportunities/fundingopportunities/bhi/sample-workplan.pdf

On Rural Evaluation Plans
Rural Health Innovations National Rural Health Resource Center. Retrieved from https://www.ruralcenter.org/rhi/network-ta/development/webinars/project-evaluation-plan-toolkit

On Conceptual Frameworks
Measure Evaluation. Family Planning and Reproductive Health Indicators Data-based. Retrieved from https://www.measureevaluation.org/prh/rh_indicators/overview/ConceptualFrameworkinRHPrograms.jpg

On Theory of Change
Center for Theory of Change. Retrieved from http://www.theoryofchange.org/what-is-theory-of-change/
United Nations Children's Fund, Theory of Change. Retrieved from http://devinfolive.info/impact_evaluation/img/downloads/Theory_of_Change_ENG.pdf

On Asset Mapping
Participatory Asset Mapping (2012). A Community Research Lab Toolkit. Retrieved from http://www.communityscience.com/knowledge4equity/AssetMappingToolkit.pdf

On Definitions for Data and Designs
Fraenkel, J. R., Wallen, N. E., & Hyun, H. H. (1993). *How to design and evaluate research in education* (Vol. 7). New York: McGraw-Hill.

On Data Collection
Center for Disease Control (2008). Data Collection Methods for Program Evaluation: Questionnaires. Retrieved from https://www.cdc.gov/healthyyouth/evaluation/pdf/brief14.pdf

Office of Research Integrity US Health and Human Services. Guidelines for Responsible Data Management in Scientific Research. Retrieved from https://ori.hhs.gov/images/ddblock/data.pdf

Rural Health Information Hub. Data Collection Strategies. Retrieved from https://www.ruralhealthinfo.org/community-health/health-promotion/4/data-collection-strategies

On Institutional Review Boards
US Department of Health and Human Services (ND). The Belmont Report. Retrieved from https://www.hhs.gov/ohrp/regulations-and-policy/belmont-report/index.html

James Bell and Associates (2008). Evaluation Brief. Understanding the Institutional Review Board January 2008. Retrieved from https://www.betterevaluation.org/sites/default/files/understanding%20the%20irb.pdf

On Sample Sizes
The Pell Institute. Determine Appropriate Sample Size Evaluation Toolkit. Retrieved from http://toolkit.pellinstitute.org/evaluation-guide/collect-data/determine-appropriate-sample-size/

On Storyboards and Logic Models
Action Evaluation Collaborative. Storyboard Activity. Retrieved from http://www.betterevaluation.org/en/resources/storyboard_activity

Chapter questions

1. Describe the five basic elements the rural evaluation process.
2. Why do you think it is important for evaluators to build trust in communities?
3. Think about a time when you really listened to someone speak. What was being said? What are some strategies to show that you are actively listening? What could happen if you were not listening?
4. List three major differences between a work plan and an evaluation plan?
5. What is an Institutional Review Board? At what point in the evaluation planning process should rural evaluators contact the IRB of record for the program/community?
6. Summarize how an evaluator might identify community resources and needs.
7. Discuss performance measures and how they are used in the evaluation plan.
8. Why is it important to have a rural evaluation plan?

Activities

1. Assume that you have been hired by a rural community school district to conduct an evaluation of a program designed to improve school attendance among K-12th graders. What is the first step that you will take as a rural community school evaluator? What are some components of the rural evaluation process that will be important to follow? What type of evaluation study design will you select? What factors should you consider when selecting an evaluation study design?
2. Select a rural community program from the Internet. Read about the program, the history, location, population, and goals and objectives. Without looking at the program's website for an evaluation plan, draft an outline of

an evaluation plan for this rural community program. What does it include? What is the purpose of the evaluation? What evaluation design did you use? What were the factors that you considered when developing the plan?

3. Design a rural program budget using the six categories outlined in this chapter. What kinds of line items are included, and what are the direct and indirect costs? What is the total program cost?

References

Ahmed, S. M., & Palermo, A. G. S. (2010). Community engagement in research: Frameworks for education and peer review. *American Journal of Public Health, 100*(8), 1380–1387.

Bickman, L. (1987). *The functions of program theory using program theory in evaluation. New directions for program evaluation* (Vol. 33). San Francisco, CA: Jossey-Bass.

Fetterman, D., & Wandersman, A. (2007). Empowerment evaluation: Yesterday, today, and tomorrow. *American Journal of Evaluation, 28*(2), 179–198.

Fitzpatrick, J. L., Sanders, J. R., & Worthen, B. R. (2004). *Program evaluation: Alternative approaches and practical guidelines.* Boston, MA: Allyn and Bacon.

Fraenkel, J. R., Wallen, N. E., & Hyun, H. H. (1993). *How to design and evaluate research in education* (Vol. 7). New York, NY: McGraw-Hill.

Jagosh, J., Bush, P. L., Salsberg, J., Macaulay, A. C., Greenhalgh, T., Wong, G. … Pluye, P. (2015). A realist evaluation of community-based participatory research: Partnership synergy, trust building and related ripple effects. *BMC Public Health, 15*(1), 725.

Jalongo, M. R. (2008). *Learning to listen, listening to learn.* Washington, DC: National Association for the Education of Young Children.

Kelley, A., Belcourt-Dittloff, A., Belcourt, C., & Belcourt, G. (2013). Research ethics and indigenous communities. *American Journal of Public Health, 103*(12), 2146–2152.

Lipsey, M. W., & Pollard, J. A. (1989). Driving toward theory in program evaluation: More models to choose from. *Evaluation and Program Planning, 12*(4), 317–328.

Mertens, D., & Hesse-Biber, S. (2013) Mixed methods and credibility of evidence in evaluation. *New Directions for Evaluation, 138*, 5–13.

Minkler, M. (2004). Ethical challenges for the "outside" researcher in community-based participatory research. *Health Education & Behavior, 31*(6), 684–697.

Patton, M. Q. (2008). *Utilization-focused evaluation.* Thousand Oaks, CA: Sage Publications.

Rogers, P. (2014). *Theory of change, methodological briefs: Impact evaluation* (Vol. 2). Florence: UNICEF Office of Research.

Rubin, R. S. (2002). Will the real SMART goals please stand up? *The Industrial-Organizational Psychologist, 39*(4), 26–27.

United States Department of Agriculture (2018). Community food systems farm to school grant program, planning grants. Retrieved from https://www.fns.usda.gov/farmtoschool/farm-school-grant-program

United States Department of Health and Human Services (ND). The Belmont Report. Retrieved from https://www.hhs.gov/ohrp/regulations-and-policy/belmont-report/index.html

Wallerstein, N. (1999). Power between evaluator and community: Research relationships within New Mexico's healthier communities. *Social Science & Medicine, 49*(1), 39–53.

6

HOW TO COLLECT AND ANALYZE DATA IN RURAL COMMUNITIES

As a rural evaluator, I find myself borrowing from both evaluation and research approaches when collecting data. I feel that evaluators are researchers and researchers are evaluators. I use many of the same data collection and analysis methods. But, I always keep the goal in mind. Is my job to find value in a program or service (evaluate) or is it to test a hypothesis, generate new knowledge, and add to the evidence base (research)? Data helps us tell the stories of what is happening in rural communities. Research helps us understand why.

Types of data used

Evaluation is driven by data. Without data, we are unable to tell the story of what is happening in rural programs and communities. In this chapter, we will become familiar with the kinds of data used in rural evaluation contexts. We have learned in the previous chapters that every community and population is unique—the kinds of data available are unique as well.

Evaluation data is generally characterized as being qualitative or quantitative in nature. **Qualitative data** is not numerical and is useful to understand the how and why of a program. In contrast, **quantitative data** is numerical and is useful for determining what is happening, how much is happening, and how much is involved. The most comprehensive evaluation includes both qualitative and quantitative data (Table 6.1).

Rural evaluators use data collection and analysis to find value, determine impact, document outcome, and cost benefit.

Process

Who do we collect data from and how is data collected? This depends on the community context, norms, goals of the program, evaluation questions, and resources available. Evaluators collect data using a variety of methods (Table 6.2).

TABLE 6.1 Types of Data

Qualitative	Quantitative
Interviews	Surveys with numeric/scaled responses
Focus groups	Parametric measures
Presentations	Scales
Written communications	Reports
Observations	Costs
Videos	
Magazines	
Art and imagery	
Photographs	
Surveys with text responses	

TABLE 6.2 How Data Are Collected

Qualitative Data Collection	Quantitative Data Collection
Interviews—Recorded and transcribed	Interviews with closed response (yes or no)—In person or via phone
Focus Groups—Recorded and transcribed	Surveys with fixed responses (A, B, C, D)—Paper, online, in person, or via phone
Filming—Taped and reviewed	Recording behaviors—Instruments or scales designed to measure
Observation—Reflection and journal notes, photographs, art, imagery, and symbols	Meta analyses—Combination of numeric results from previous programs or efforts
Surveys with open text response—Transcribed and analyzed	Existing numeric data (population characteristics, income, demographics, health disparities, education statistics, unemployment)

When and where?

Data is collected based on time, population or group of interest, and geographic area. Time refers to the period of time for which the evaluation is focused. Groups of interest may include families, livestock owners, participants in a program, and trainees who are located in a geographic area at a time of interest. Geographic areas may include a town, county, or region (Taylor-Powell, 1998).

Who collects data?

Program evaluators, community members, program leads, and recipients of programs being implemented may collect data. Often evaluators collect data in rural communities. When evaluators collect data for evaluation purposes, this often results in information about the program, the intervention, and the outcome, from the perspective of the evaluator. However, the increase of participatory evaluation strategies such as utilization-focused evaluation and empowerment evaluation have increased the number of non-evaluators collecting data.

How much?

The amount of data that you need to collect depends on the purpose of the evaluation, the data available, and how these data document the outcome. With quantitative data, consider the selection of people, activities, actions, and other inputs for the program. Then determine the sample size needed. You may estimate the sample size based on a proportion, based on a mean for a specific population or a variable of interest, or by using a finite population correction factor when the sample is over 5 percent of the proportion of the population (Rose, Spinks, & Canhoto, 2015). The amount of qualitative data needed varies. Guest and colleagues reviewed 60 interviews and found that most qualitative codes emerged in the first 12 interviews (2006). Lasch and colleagues recommend focus groups with 6–12 people (2010). The amount of data is not the point, but rather the quality of data and its ability to answer the evaluation question at hand. Ultimately, evaluators should try to collect enough data to reach saturation, meaning a rich and thick description of the evaluand.

One of the most important things to remember when collecting data is that we must be ethical in how we collect it. That means that we are respectful, we ensure confidentiality if the conditions require it, and we follow local, state, and funding agency ethical guidelines.

Develop and pilot evaluation instruments

An **evaluation instrument** is anything that is used to collect the information that is needed in the evaluation. Examples of evaluation instruments may include a Likert-type scale developed to assess community satisfaction with a program's service or a video recording of an interview. Box 6.1.

There are many different evaluation instruments available—do not feel overwhelmed because in the next section we are going to review some guidelines for how to select a method for collecting evaluation data.

Evaluators pilot instruments to establish their reliability and validity. **Instrument reliability** is the ability of an instrument to repeatedly produce the same results. **Instrument validity** refers to the degree to which an instrument measures what it is supposed to measure (Trochim, 2006). **External validity** is the degree to which findings from an instrument/data collected can be generalized from a sample to a population (Mertens, 2014). **Content validity** is the degree to which an instrument measures and collects content that evaluators need to know. These terms apply to both qualitative and quantitative data (Golafshani, 2003). Imagine creating a questionnaire without paying attention to the population that will be completing it. If the questionnaire is to be completed by

---

BOX 6.1 Field notes on evaluation instruments

Over the years, I have used a lot of different evaluation instruments. I recall that early in my career, I would attend meetings, conferences, or presentations and listen. I might take notes and even a few photos, but I never recorded anything that anyone said on paper, word-for-word. Several years passed and reports were generated using a variety of evaluation instruments. Then, one day I realized that some of the most valuable information that I needed to know for the evaluation was not included on the evaluation instruments. The message from speakers and the audience was what I needed to capture. I needed to know what things presenters were sharing and how the audience responded to these topics, with questions, or silence in some cases.

Recording and observing in these exchanges in an ethical manner has been a powerful way to enhance evaluation findings in rural communities.

---

second graders, but uses a fifth-grade reading level, the data resulting from this questionnaire will not be very credible. If you are unsure of the literacy level of a population you will be working with, make sure you pilot the evaluation instruments first. For more information on literacy levels and assessing evaluation instruments to ensure they are at the correct literacy level, read the additional resources section at the end of this chapter.

Review results and refine process

If you are new to a program or community, it may take some time to know what kinds of evaluation instruments are most responsive to the needs of the community. In some communities, videotaping and recording are not normative. However, in other instances videotaping and recording may be perfectly acceptable. When you select an evaluation instrument, make sure that it is acceptable to the community. Test the evaluation instrument and do not be afraid to abandon one evaluation instrument, and move to another. Evaluation in rural communities requires flexibility and understanding that what works in some communities may not work in others, or what worked a year ago might not work today.

Credible evidence

Credible evidence in evaluation considers the community context, logistics, indicators, evaluation instruments, and the quality and quantity of data that evaluation instruments produce.

Once you have piloted your evaluation instrument and you feel confident that it will produce credible results, it is time to revisit the program goals and evaluation questions. Are there questions that you included in the initial piloting process that you do not feel are necessary? Is the evaluation instrument too long? Are the questions sensitive to the needs of the community? Is it acceptable to videotape or record in the community setting or with the population? Will the instrument produce the kinds of results that funding agencies, policy makers, and communities need?

Use various data sources

Rural America is characterized by a small population (<2,500 people) and because of this, selecting an appropriate data collection strategy is extremely important. Luckily we have primary and secondary data sources to help us as evaluators. We know from earlier chapters that **primary data** collection sources include surveys, interviews, focus groups, document reviews, meeting minutes, and more. **Secondary data** sources are those which already exist. In rural communities, these include the United States Census data, state vital statistics, various national and state surveillance databases, and United States Department of Agriculture (USDA) Economic Research Service. The use of primary or secondary data sources in evaluation depends on a number of different factors.

Data sources

Primary data

Using primary data in rural evaluation is helpful because evaluation instruments can be designed to answer a specific evaluation question. Evaluators can ensure that appropriate evaluation instruments are selected and appropriate for the population and context. However, primary data collection can also be challenging in rural evaluation contexts. Consider the expense of collecting data—this often requires travel to the community, preparing instruments, collecting the data, and analyzing the data.

Secondary data

Using secondary data in rural evaluation can be useful. Knowing what data sets are available and how to access these data are extremely important. The main benefit of using secondary data in evaluation is that it is available now, and it does not require any data collection on your part. Secondary data is also inexpensive—most secondary data sets are free and available to the public.

Administrative data is another type of secondary data. Administrative data is collected by an organization or business that is part of daily operations. Examples of administrative data include hospital intake and discharge records, employee records, traffic violations, daily sales, and more. The advantages of using administrative data are: it is free, it often includes a large number of data points that can be viewed over time, and it is updated regularly (Table 6.3).

TABLE 6.3 Advantages and Disadvantages of Primary, Secondary, and Administrative Data

Data Type	Advantage	Disadvantage
Primary data	Collected for the purposes of the evaluation to answer specific questions, recent data, source is known	Expensive. Takes time. Some people may not want to participate. Requires trained data collectors and trained developers of instruments. Respondents may not respond truthfully. May not be generalizable to other populations. May only reflect a small sample of the population.
Secondary data	Inexpensive, data is already collected, useful for documenting current needs and resources available, and can be combined with other data sources	May not include all outcomes of interest or address the evaluation question(s). May not include dates of interest. Missing data is common. Rural communities may not be captured, may lack comparison data.
Administrative data	Lots of information, updated consistently, readability available, more accurate than self-report, inexpensive	No control over data collected, instrument used, outcomes reported. Missing cases, data entry errors, and differences in data types make it difficult to compare or analyze.

Quantitative data collection methods

Quantitative data collection methods include any method that results in a response that is or can be transformed into a number. Quantitative data answers questions like, "How many?", "Who was involved?", "What was the outcome?", "How much did it cost?", and "What changed?" (Agency for Toxic Substance Disease Registry15.2, 2015). There are two types of quantitative data that rural evaluators may encounter: discrete and continuous. **Discrete data** is that which has a set number of values. Examples of discrete data include tests with a set number of questions, or survey data that asks the number of cars a family owns. In contrast, **continuous data** is that which falls on a continuum. Examples of continuous data include height, age, weight, or distance (Creswell & Creswell, 2017). Quantitative data may be collected using observation, document review, patient chart review, observation, or data collected during a pre- or posttest. Forms may report quantitative data and are often used in evaluation (Krueger, 2017). Examples include an adult physical where height, weight, blood pressure, and cholesterol are collected. Other forms may include observations, checklists, costs, or interviews where responses are numeric. Surveys can be quantitative as well. **Surveys** are structured questionnaires used to generate quantitative or qualitative data. Surveys can either be paper or electronic and completed by an individual in person, over the phone, or using the

---

BOX 6.2 Probability sampling formula

N = the number of cases in the sampling frame
n = the number of cases in the sample
nCn = the number of combinations of n from N
f = the sampling fraction n/N
An example of a sampling frame of 1,000 people with 100 people selected
$f = n/N = 100/1000 = .10$ or 10%

Source: Adapted from the Web Center for Social Research
Methods (2006). Probability Sampling. Retrieved from https://www.
socialresearchmethods.net/kb/sampprob.php

Internet. To know how many quantitative surveys are needed to generalize findings to the larger population, evaluators use probability sampling. **Probability sampling** is any sampling method that includes random selection (Box 6.2). The most common form of probability sampling in rural evaluation contexts is simple random sampling. The objective of simple random sampling is to select individuals out of a population in such a way that all have an equal chance of being selected.

Qualitative data collection methods

Qualitative data methods answer questions like, "What is the value?", "What happened?", and "How did people feel?" (ATSDR, 2015). Qualitative data may be collected via forms, surveys, or questionnaires using open-text response. For example, "What was the best part of the training today?" Responses are typed or written using their own words. **Interviews** are another form of qualitative data and are helpful in documenting perspectives, experiences, and ideas about a given project or context (Manzano, 2016). Interviews may take place with individuals, one-on-one, or in a group setting (focus group). When preparing for an interview, consider the three types of interviews: structured, semistructured, or unstructured. **Structured interviews** are typically used in evaluations when responses are established already; respondents select from a list of preestablished answers rather than open-ended questions. Questions are asked in a specific order and the approach is focused and rigid. **Semistructured interviews** are often developed based on a guiding theme or principle that is underpinning an evaluation. Semistructured interviews may include yes or no responses along with open-ended responses. Evaluators working in rural communities often use semistructured interviews because they allow more flexibility and changing or leaving questions out based on context. The last type of interview is unstructured. **Unstructured interviews** are just that; they are conversations about

---

BOX 6.3 Field notes on focus groups

We facilitated a focus group with 12 middle school boys from a rural community. Our goal was to learn more about the kinds of activities they would like to have in their community. It did not work as planned. The boys did not respond to the questions, and in some cases the questions were not clear, or they did not know how to respond. This resulted in data that was not complete, and a lack of understanding about what kinds of activities that kids want in their community. When facilitating a focus group, know your audience, think about different ways to ask the question, and consider semistructured interviews or other data collection methods when working with specific topics and populations.

---

what is happening and discussions are not based on an established theme or set of questions, but rather what individuals feel is most important to discuss (Kelley, MedicineBull, LaFranier, 2016). **Digital storytelling** data uses images and narratives developed by community members or participant groups to describe a phenomenon of interest (Gubrium & Turner, 2011). Data from digital stories can be analyzed and used by rural evaluators to describe, explain, or transform areas of interest. **Focus Groups** are a discussion among a group of people about a specific issue. Focus groups are useful when evaluators want to know the attitudes, beliefs, or issues of a specific group. Focus groups are also useful for establishing a program to address a particular need, or to build on existing program efforts and support further work. Focus groups require time, a skilled moderator, and a set of questions. Questions are developed by the evaluator and in conjunction with community, program staff, and other stakeholders. Generally, focus groups are homogenous, that is, a group of people with similar backgrounds, perspectives, or a unifying interest. Most often focus groups include 8–12 people and discussions are often videotaped or recorded for transcription and analyses (Box 6.3).

Other data collection methods and sources

Funding agency reports and grant proposals

Information submitted to the funding agency by the community can be useful data source for rural evaluators. Typically funding agencies require quarterly or annual reports. These reports are populated by data that comes from primary, secondary, or administrative data sources. Because each funding agency has a separate set of guidelines for reporting, evaluators need to be familiar with these guidelines early, understand how they are reported, and how existing data from the evaluation plan can be used to populate funding agency requirements (Box 6.4).

BOX 6.4 Field notes on multiple data sources for meeting funding agency reporting requirements

I have been working with six rural communities for four years. These communities are part of a consortium effort to reduce substance use in youth. Each community has a site coordinator who is responsible for implementing a variety of prevention activities. These activities are then reported to the facilitating agency. I receive activity sheets and invoices quarterly. As the lead evaluator I then analyze all data using a mixed-methods approach (because I have both qualitative and quantitative data). After I analyze all of the mixed data, I enter the data and themes into the funding agency online reporting system.

I use program budgets (administrative data) to report on the funds allocated for prevention activities and the funds spent to date, and how these funds are allocated for each of the established goals.

This process takes a lot of time, but after four years of working on the project I have come to realize that it is the only way to get the data that is needed to satisfy the funding agency requirements. Developing new forms, tools, even scheduling interviews with site coordinators did not work. The addition of more paperwork and tasks to complete for the evaluation was not welcomed. We decided that the best way to move forward was to use data that has already been collected.

Observations

One of the best ways to understand what is happening in a rural program is to observe. This requires presence in the community, and relationship with the community. Observers are trained, prepared, and systematic in their approach (Krueger, 2017). Observations are useful when you are wanting to see how people interact with one another, you want to know how a process works, you want to know the behaviors of a specific group, you want to see how people behave in a meeting or public event, you want to know if people follow laws, rules, or guidelines, or you want to know if behaviors have changed as a result of a program or intervention. Observation data may be collected using field notes, memos, or checklists.

News and Internet

Data sources found on the Internet and local news can be useful. These secondary data sources may be qualitative, quantitative, or mixed and provide information on context, up-to-date information on current events, and other information that may be useful. News and Internet data sources may include write-ups on a community or program, a press release on funding or award, information about upcoming meetings and locations, photographs of interventions that are occurring in a community as a result of a program, or even information that documents the need for future programming and services.

One recent topic that is making the news in rural America is the opioid epidemic. Rural Americans experience disproportionate rates of opioid use and opioid mortality than other Americans (Box 6.5).

When using news and Internet sources as data in rural evaluation, make sure the data are credible and accurate. There are several guides to evaluating Internet resources available. Consider the author, purpose, objectivity, accuracy, reliability and credibility, how current the information is, and the links associated with the site. For more information on evaluating Internet articles, review the additional resources section at the end of this chapter.

BOX 6.5 Rural opioid epidemic web-based news article excerpt

SALT LAKE CITY, Utah (News4Utah)—It's deemed one of the biggest health crises of our time.

The opioid epidemic is a problem that's plaguing rural communities across the nation. So much so that the United States Department of Agriculture (USDA) is partnering with rural leaders to address the crisis through regional roundtable discussions. Wednesday, Anne Hazlett, the USDA's Assistant to the Secretary for Rural Development joined federal, state and local leaders at the Utah State Capitol for one of these discussions. They joined forces with eleven panelists who work in the field of prevention to tackle the problem head on. "We must accept change. We must start thinking outside the box with prevention and resources," one of the panelists said. According to the Center of Disease Control and Prevention, Utah has one of the highest death rates due to drug overdose. In 2016, the state lost 635 people to this epidemic. "The opioid epidemic in rural communities is more than a public health issue," Hazlett said. "This is a matter of rural prosperity. Opioid misuse is impacting the quality of life and economic well-being in small towns," she added. The main goals of the discussion was how to spread awareness about this issue in rural Utah, catch greedy dealers, and ultimately save lives. The issue is these drug traffickers aren't just on the streets. Sometimes, they are trusted doctors.

Source: Good4Utah Local News. USDA Hosts roundtable focused on the opioid epidemic in rural Utah April 12, 2018 by Jen Jacobson. Retrieved from http://www.good4utah.com/news/local-news/roundtable-focuses-on-opioid-epidemic-in-utah/1117341054

Data quality

We know that evaluation data must be accurate and reliable. **Accurate** information is correct and represents the truth about what we intend to measure. **Reliable** information is collected and measured consistently using quality measures. Evaluators can help ensure reliable data collection using consistent measures and approaches to collect data throughout a program. In rural communities, activities may be implemented as part of a program and these activities often produce measurable results. A rural evaluator supports communities by collecting and recording results in a systematic way.

Factors that may affect data quality in rural evaluation contexts may include programmatic, measurement, and instrumentation factors. **Programmatic data quality** relates to changes in how a program is implemented. For example, changes to staffing, program activities, and outreach would likely increase or decrease program activity and the subsequent results. **Measurement factors** related to data quality include changes in how activities are defined and supported. These changes may result in differences in results reported over time. When we change definitions, key terms, or approaches, direct comparison can be difficult. **Instrumentation factors** relate to data quality and how data are collected. Sometimes people refer to this as instrumentation bias. When we change instruments, it is nearly impossible to compare evaluation results (Box 6.6).

BOX 6.6 Field notes on instrumentation factors

We developed an instrument to assess changes in youth-perceived risk related to substance use. We piloted the instrument with youth and had several people review the instrument.

Several months into the intervention, we noticed that the response options for some of the questions were not complete. This was a question and the original survey response options:

1. How much are people at risk for harming themselves if they drink five or more alcohol beverages once or twice a week?
   a No risk
   b Slight risk
   c Great risk
   d Don't know

In the response options we omitted moderate risk. This resulted in a 3-point scale rather than a 4-point scale and unequal intervals between categories. We added moderate risk to the survey after we noticed our mistake, but direct comparison of this survey question was not possible because we changed the response options.

Many of the data analyses approaches summarized in the next section are based on scientific methods and evaluation research strategies. Your approach to evaluating data will largely depend on the questions that your evaluation seeks to answer and the approach that is used to arrive at these answers.

> Evaluation research means supplying valid and reliable evidence regarding the operation of social programs or clinical practices—how they are planned, how well they operate, and how effectively they achieve their goals.
>
> —*(Monette, Sullivan, & DeJong, 1990, p. 337)*

Preparing the data

Data preparation begins after data is collected. Sometimes this involves reviewing the data, counting data, checking the data to make sure it is accurate, logging the information, entering the data into a computer, or uploading data. Rural evaluators may receive data in the form of photos, surveys, observations, videos, drawings, administrative data, and a variety of other sources. Trochim (2006) recommends a six-step process for preparing data: log data, check for accuracy, develop a database, enter data into a computer, transform data, and prepare to analyze data.

Data analysis

Analyzing data as rural evaluators is one of the most important aspects of our profession. Planning for data analysis should begin before you collect any data. Data analysis plans can be extremely helpful. A **data analysis plan** is a roadmap for how you will analyze your data (see Appendix B). These plans begin with identifying what data need to be collected and end with collecting and managing data. Visual descriptions link program components, tasks, outcomes, measures, and analytic approaches to be used in the data analysis planning process (Table 6.4).

A note on measures, they can be nominal, scale, ratio, or ordinal. **Nominal data** refers to measures that use a description or classification. **Interval data** measures in equal intervals but does not have an absolute zero. Likert scale rankings are one example where 1 is very dissatisfied and 5 is very satisfied. **Ratio data** is continuous with equal differences between values, with an absolute zero. Height, weight, and age are examples of ratio data. Ordinal data does not have an absolute zero, and rank order is one example. These classifications help the software know what the data are, beyond a number or a name. Once you have identified measures that will be used in the rural evaluation process, create a table that outlines the measures, source, frequency, method, and level of data (Table 6.5).

There are different approaches for analyzing data depending on the kinds of data that you collect.

TABLE 6.4 Field Notes on Evaluative Aims and Analysis Methods

Program Component	Program Tasks	Expected Outcome	Process or Outcome Measure /Frequency	Analytic Approach
Aim 1: To monitor and assess the number of individuals reached through the substance use prevention program in six rural communities.				
Alcohol- and drug-free activities	Plan and implement cultural and educational events for youth	1,200 youth participate and complete participant surveys.	Number of participants Participant survey	Descriptive statistics
Aim 2: To monitor and assess self-reported underage drinking in six rural communities.				
Program Component	Program Tasks	Expected Outcome	Process or Outcome Measure	Analytic Approach
Prevention messages, trainings, and education	Identify baseline data from Youth Risk Factor Behavior Survey (YRBS) for each community.	Reduce self-reported underage drinking in the past 30 days by 30%	Reduction in underage drinking after involvement in program activities Participant survey	t-test, correlation, and multiple regression

TABLE 6.5 Field Notes on Measures, Frequency Source, Method, and Level of Data

Measure	Source	Frequency	Method	Level of Data
Thirty-day alcohol	YRBS	Annually	Administrative	County
Thirty-day prescription drug misuse	YRBS	Annually	Administrative	County
Two-week binge drink	YRBS	Annually	Administrative	County
Perception of parental disapproval and attitude	PNA	Annually	Administrative	County

YRBS=Youth Risk Factor Behavior Survey.
PNA=Prevention Needs Assessment.

Analyzing quantitative data

Quantitative data deals with numbers. There are some common terms related to quantitative data analysis that you should definitely know. A **statistic** is a number that is used to describe a sample characteristic. **Data** is a characteristic or number. A **population** is a complete set of actual or potential observations. A **parameter** is a number that describes a population characteristic, often referred to as a sample statistic. A **sample** is a subset of the population that is intentionally selected. A **random sample** is a subset of a sample that is selected in a manner that is random, that is every member of the population has an equal chance of being selected. **A variable** is a term used to describe a data point that is being collected in the evaluation. Variables can take on different values and may include age, gender, a specific activity, or a treatment group (Simpson, 2015). There are three types of variable analysis: univariate, bivariate, and multivariate. Univariate involves just one variable, for example, age. Bivariate involves two variables, for example, age and gender. Multivariate involves more than two variables. A value is related to a variable and further defines it, for example, the values for gender are male or female (Box 6.7).

Approaches used to analyze quantitative data vary depending on the data that you have and the evaluation questions that you want to answer with your data.

BOX 6.7 Field notes on univariate and bivariate outputs

Univariate Output, Gender Is the only Variable

		Frequency	Percent	Valid Percent	Cumulative Percent
Valid	Male	245	42.5	42.5	42.5
	Female	331	57.5	57.5	100.0
	Total	576	100.0	100.0	

Bivariate Output with Gender and Age

		Gender		Total
		Male	Female	
Age	12	35	45	80
	13	48	66	114
	13.5	1	0	1
	14	52	90	142
	15	45	65	110
	16	26	28	54
	17	21	16	37
	18	10	10	20
	19	2	3	5
	20	1	1	2
Mean Age (SD)		14.4 years (SD=1.74)	14.3 years (SD=1.59)	14.3 years (SD=1.66)
Total		241	324	565

Previous authors describe two basic types of quantitative data analysis tools: descriptive and inferential. **Descriptive data** simply describes data using several different tools: the mean, median, mode, frequency distribution, standard deviation, and variance analysis. **Inferential data** is used to make generalizations about a population from which the sample was taken. Tools used to achieve inference include t-tests, analysis of variance (ANOVA), hypothesis testing, Chi-square, regression, correlation, and z-scores.

The total sample of a population is referred to using N and a subgroup within a population is referred to as n. Wilcox et al. (2000) provide the following example, "Rural ($n = 1242$) and urban ($n = 1096$) women aged 40 years and older from the US Women's Determinants Study" (para. 3).

Descriptive data may include mean and standard deviation. Where M represents the **mean** or the average value of a sample or population and SD represents the **standard deviation** or the square root of the variance. **Variance** is the average of square differences between observations and their means.

Statistical significance is used to determine if there are differences in an outcome due to chance. Most often significance levels are set at (p) .95. This means that there is a 95% chance that the results are true or $1 - p$. Significance is reported using (p) .001 or .05, and these numbers mean that there is a .001% or 5% chance that the results are not true (Rice, 1989). Different statistical tests will report p values for you to consider. **Hypotheses testing** relates to the significance levels above and is used to test ideas about a group or population. There is a null hypothesis (H_0) and an alternative hypothesis (H_1). The null hypothesis is a statement that we assume to be true. The alternative hypothesis (H_1) is used when we reject the null hypothesis and find the alternate hypothesis to be true. Alpha (α) is the lowest level that can be used to reject the null hypothesis. There are Type I errors and Type II errors, where evaluators reject the null hypothesis, even if it is true or correct. For more information on hypothesis testing, review the resources section at the end of this chapter.

Chi-square tests are used to compare two groups of categorical data (data that can be counted or grouped into categories). The Chi-square test is noted by the X^2 symbol and is used to measure the distribution of data and values. Wilcox et al. compared rural and urban women who were sedentary, without a high school education, "X^2 (1, $N = 394$) $= 8.87$, $p = .001$" (2000, p. 669), where (1, $N = 394$) represents the degrees of freedom, 8.87 represents the Pearson Chi-square value, and p represents the significance level. The Chi-square statistic of 8.87 is used to calculate the p value.

t-**Tests** are used to answer the question, "Is the difference between two samples different (significant) enough to say that something else could have caused the difference?" Kahn (2010) provides the following example of a t-test, "There was a significant effect for gender, t (54) $= 5.43$, $p < .001$, with men receiving higher scores than women" (2010, para. 4), where t indicates that a t-test was conducted, (54) represents the degrees of freedom, 5.43 is the result of the calculation/t-statistic, and $p < .001$ is the probability that the difference is significant.

Remember that if you are examining matched groups, a *t*-test for correlated samples is used (Mertens, 2014).

Correlation analyses are used to describe the strength and linear relationship between two variables. The *r* value will always be between +1 and −1, where −1.00 represents a perfect negative linear relationship and +1.00 represents a perfect positive linear relationship. Deborah Rumsey and Unger (2015) describe these values using a hill, where −1.00 is a perfect downhill slope and +1.0 is a perfect uphill slope. Wilcox, et al. (2000) explored the correlations between independent variables to describe relationships between race and neighborhood location. "Hispanic race was related to living in the West ($r = .45$, $p < .001$). African American race was negatively related to the presence of sidewalks in one's neighborhood ($r = −.34$, $p < .001$)" (p. 670). The *r* represents the correlation coefficient and the negative *r* value of −.34 indicates a weak negative (or downhill) relationship between African American race and sidewalks and the *r* value of .45 shows a weak to moderate positive (uphill) relationship between Hispanic race and those living in the West (Wilcox, et al., 2000).

ANOVA can be helpful in determining if there is a statistically significant difference between three or more groups based on mean scores. ANOVAs are used to determine the mean of an intervention or experimental treatment. The main utility of ANOVA in rural evaluation is to compare how much one might expect means to spread out if all groups were sampled from the same population, and there were no population differences (Rumsey & Unger, 2015). Kahn provides the following example of an ANOVA, "There was a significant main effect for treatment, $F(1, 145) = 5.43$, $p = .02$, and a significant interaction, $F(2, 145) = 3.24$, $p = .04$" (2010, para. 5). ANOVAs result in a *t*-test statistic called the *F*-ratio. *F* represents the variability between and within groups or degrees of freedom between and within groups.

Other inferential statistic methods include analysis of covariance, regression analyses, factor analysis, multidimensional scaling, cluster analysis, and many others (Trochim, 2006). These analyses require specific computer software and a more advanced understanding of statistics.

Descriptive statistics are commonly used in rural program evaluation. These include frequency distributions, percent distributions, mean, median, mode, maximum and minimum values mentioned at the beginning of this section. However, the evaluation questions and the data collected will determine the kinds of analyses that are appropriate. But how do we know that the quantitative data is valid and reliable?

Quantitative validity and reliability

Validity is ensuring that a test measures what it aims to measure. There are four types of validity commonly used: conclusion validity, internal validity, construct validity, and external validity (Hernon & Schwartz, 2009). **Conclusion validity** seeks to establish a relationship between the program/intervention and outcome. **Internal validity** seeks to document the relationship between the program/intervention and the outcome observed based on a causal relationship. **Construct validity** seeks to determine the degree to which a test or question measures what it is supposed to measure. **External validity** seeks to generalize results from one evaluation or study to another. **Quantitative reliability** refers to the consistency of a measure to produce the same results with the same people, under the same conditions (Hernon & Schwartz, 2009). Test–retest and internal consistency are two methods for documenting reliability with quantitative data.

Qualitative data analysis

Qualitative data deals with information that is not in numeric form. Unlike quantitative data analyses described in the previous section, qualitative data analyses are subjective and are based on interpretation (Creswell & Creswell, 2017). Similar to quantitative analyses, we begin with a data analysis plan. A qualitative data analysis plan includes the primary evaluation question(s), identifying the individual(s) that will enter and analyze the data, knowing how much data you plan to collect, and identifying what tools you will need to analyze the data.

Four qualitative approaches

There are four primary approaches in qualitative analyses: a general inductive approach, grounded theory, discourse analysis, and phenomenology (Thomas, 2006). Evaluators often select an approach based on a paradigm. Schwandt defines paradigm as a shared worldview that represents the beliefs and values in a discipline that guide how we approach and solve problems (2001).

Inductive analysis is an approach that uses raw data to create concepts, themes, or conceptual models based on an evaluators interpretation of data (Thomas, 2006). Inductive analysis begins within a general area of study. Theories emerge from the data. Thomas recommends three instances when the inductive approach is appropriate: (1) to condense raw data into a brief summary, (2) to document links between evaluation objectives and findings, and (3) to develop a model or theory about what is occurring based on the data (2006). Characteristics of inductive analysis include category labels, category descriptions, text with categories, links, and models or frameworks (Thomas, 2006).

Grounded theory data analysis involves open coding of text with the goal of developing a theoretical framework (Glaser & Strauss, 1967). Grounded theory comes from the field of sociology and its goal is to develop an explanatory theory of a social process. An example question that grounded theory could answer is, "How does the basic social process of [X] happen in the context of [Y] environment?" (Starks & Trinidad, 2007, p. 1373).

Discourse analysis is used to understand how language creates and supports identities and events (Wodak & Meyer, 2009). Discourse analysis comes from the field of linguistics. An example question that discourse analysis could answer is, "What discourses are used and how do they shape identities, activities, and relationships?" (Starks & Trinidad, 2007, p. 1373). Discourse analysis may be useful in understanding rural communities, their discourse (language), and how discourse shapes their identity and relationships.

Phenomenology is used to describe the meaning of a phenomenon based on a lived experience (Charmaz & McMullen, 2011). An example question that phenomenology could answer is, "What is the lived experience of the [phenomenon of interest]?" (Starks & Trinidad, 2007, p. 1373).

Other qualitative approaches include deductive analysis, narrative analysis, intuitive inquiry, and ethnographic analysis. When selecting a qualitative approach, know the questions you want answered, the context, and the meaning.

Once you have established a qualitative data analysis plan and selected an approach, you can analyze the data. There are several qualitative analysis software programs available (see Table 6.6). Analyzing qualitative data begins with a review of the different kinds of data that you have. After the review, organize database on the evaluation questions that you want to answer. If you conducted a focus group to explore youth perceptions of substance use in rural America, you might begin with transcribing your notes or audio recording. You might also have photographs from the focus groups, a diagram of how the room or tables were set up, and the position of the facilitator in relation to the participants. Other data may be notes, observations, a journal, activity log, agenda, and grant documents or reports. Once you have organized all of your data, it is time to analyze the data. Determine which data you will use. Sometimes we collect so much qualitative data it feels overwhelming; but, do not feel that way, focus on the primary evaluation question that the qualitative data can answer.

Analytic methods in qualitative approaches use a variety of techniques. These techniques are often derived from the qualitative approach and supported by the existing literature. **Analytic methods** may include coding, sorting, identifying themes, establishing relationships between variables, and drawing conclusions (Starks & Trinidad, 2007). **Content analysis** is a process of finding meaning from the content of the data, and it allows for flexibility in the approach and procedures used to analyze data. Hsieh and Shannon provide more information in their publication, *Three Approaches to Qualitative Content Analysis Content* (2005). Box 6.8 provides an example of how to approach qualitative data analysis.

Coding is a process of identifying short text or phrases in your data that correspond to the evaluation question. **Categories** may be used to group coded segments, for example, rural towns is the category and the coded text are the Colorado towns of Yuma, Otis, and Brush. **Themes** build on categories and relate to the evaluation question, for example, limited access to health care in rural Colorado towns. A common qualitative data analysis method used in rural evaluation is content analysis.

BOX 6.8 Field notes on qualitative data analysis

1. Read and review all data.
2. Identify key concepts, ideas, and themes.
3. Define and code important ideas and themes in a codebook, either as they emerge or based on evaluation focus or theory.
4. Code the data with at least two independent coders:
   - i   This can be done either by hand or using software.
   - ii   If you are just starting or have a small number of documents to examine, code text by hand.
   - iii If you have multiple documents and types (i.e. posters, poems, photographs, and videos), qualitative software programs allow you to import, code, and visualize data.
5. Summarize the coded data:
   - i   Look for patterns and relationships among themes.
   - ii   Identify how often themes occur in the context.
   - iii Refer back to field notes, evaluation plan, emails, and other information to clarify.
6. Pull out quotes or exemplars of themes as they emerge.
   Additional data steps

   - i   Create codebook and test it.
   - ii   Intra- or inter-coder reliability.
   - iii Recode if there are discrepancies.
   - iv   Identify how consistent the data are.
   - v   Examine the themes and their relationship to each other.
   - vi   Finalize data in a format that is most useful to the community/purpose.
   - vii Share results.

Thematic data analysis is used when the interest is exploring themes or patterns in and across data, and the visual representation of themes and the relationships between them (Attride-Stirling, 2001). Figure 6.1 displays community and stakeholder perspectives of the mental health system, with three themes that describe history, resources, and recommendations, broad categories, and coded text.

Once everything is coded, it is time to interpret. Interpreting data can feel intimidating because it is subjective in nature, and it includes your experiences, perceptions, and those of the community. Interpreting data is an iterative, inductive process that decontextualizes data for the context and evaluation purpose. When interpreting the results, consider the evaluation purpose, the evaluation question(s), and the audience.

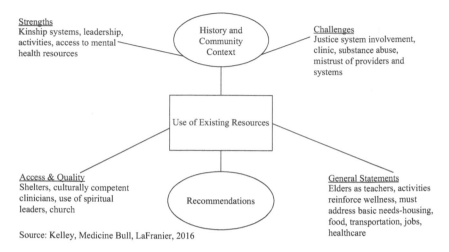

Strengths
Kinship systems, leadership, activities, access to mental health resources

History and Community Context

Challenges
Justice system involvement, clinic, substance abuse, mistrust of providers and systems

Use of Existing Resources

Access & Quality
Shelters, culturally competent clinicians, use of spiritual leaders, church

Recommendations

General Statements
Elders as teachers, activities reinforce wellness, must address basic needs-housing, food, transportation, jobs, healthcare

Source: Kelley, Medicine Bull, LaFranier, 2016

FIGURE 6.1 Thematic Analysis Systems of Care Rural Evaluation.

Triangulation
• Use multiple sources of information to create themes or categories in a study.

Member Checking
• Present results to participants in the program to confirm credibility

Engagement in the Field
• Evaluators spend time in community, observe, compare, relate, and understand context.

Collaboration
• Evaluator works with community, builds community perspectives and values in qualitative approach

Documentation
• Evaluator keeps a log of activities, data collection times and locations, and data analyses procedures.

Rich Description
• A narrative account of what is occurring in the program or community that highlights how people feel, their relationships, and interactions.

Peer Debriefing
• External review of the evaluation data and findings by someone knowledgeable about the focus but not involved in the evaluation or program.

Source: Adapted from Creswell, J. W., & Miller, D. L. (2000).

FIGURE 6.2 Seven Factors that Determine Validity of Qualitative Data.

Qualitative validity

In the last decade, there has been an increase in the use of qualitative data analysis methods (Creswell & Creswell, 2017; Creswell & Miller, 2000). However, some evaluators are concerned with the validity of qualitative data analysis. Guba and Lincoln identified specific threats to qualitative data: use of multiple perspectives to document truth, issues with dependability, application of results to other contexts and populations, and bias introduced by the evaluator/researcher (1989). Factors that determine validity of qualitative data should be considered early in the data analysis process (Figure 6.2).

Mixed methods data analysis

Mixed-methods analyses involve both qualitative and quantitative data. There is a long history of mixed-methods research that came from the fields of social, behavioral, and human science disciplines. In the early 1950s and 1960s, the only people using mixed-methods research were sociologists (Johnson, Onwuegbuzie, & Turner, 2007).

The procedures we discussed earlier to analyze qualitative and quantitative data should be applied in mixed-methods data analysis. However, because mixed methods involve two kinds of data, it is important to identify how the data will be transformed and analyzed and at what point this will occur in the evaluation process. One common mixed-methods approach is transforming data. One example of data transformation is coding qualitative data and counting the number of times that codes and themes appear in the data (Creswell & Creswell, 2017). Another example of mixed-methods analyses in evaluation is supporting quantitative data with qualitative data. Perhaps the quantitative data collected in an evaluation does not make sense. Interviews with survey respondents could help clarify the data and why they are different from the rest of the sample.

Mixed-methods validity

Validity procedures in mixed-methods data analysis are also important. These procedures involve reviewing quantitative and qualitative data for accuracy and triangulating data sources when appropriate (Creswell & Creswell, 2017) (Figure 6.3).

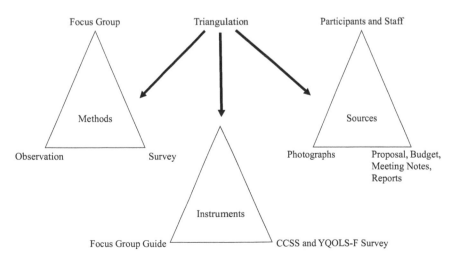

FIGURE 6.3   Field Notes on Triangulating Data.

Software

The car sits in the garage because nobody knows how to drive it

Software is helpful for analyzing all types of data. Some rural communities may not have access to a computer, and others may not have the computer skills necessary to utilize the various software programs available. When engaging community in the rural evaluation data analysis process, consider technology access, computer skills, statistical skills, and the budget available. Below are some software programs that rural evaluators use (Table 6.6).

In the last decade, the use of online or web-based surveys has increased (Wright, 2005); however, sampling bias along with access issues are problematic, especially in rural America. According to Wright, there were over 20 different web survey companies (2005). The cost of using web-based surveys varies based on intended use, features, and services provided. Other computer programs that are used by rural evaluators include Microsoft products like Excel, PowerPoint, Access, and Publisher.

Learnings. Limitations. Assumptions from the data

All data that we collect as evaluators has something to tell us. There are limitations to every data set that relate to how data were collected, a small sample size, selection bias, or the currency of the data. Knowing these limitations and revisiting them in the evaluation process is what effective rural evaluators do. We can also make assumptions based on the data. In qualitative evaluation approaches, we make assumptions in order to develop theories and concepts, and find meaning.

TABLE 6.6 Field Notes on Qualitative and Quantitative Software Programs

Qualitative Software	*Quantitative Software*
NVivo, QSR International (see, www.qsrinternational.com/nvivo/nvivo-products	IBM SPSS (see, www.ibm.com/products/spss-statistics/pricing)
QDA miner and QDA miner lite (see https://provalisresearch.com/products/qualitative-data-analysis-software/)	STATA (see www.stata.com/)
ATLAS.ti (see https://atlasti.com/)	SAS (see www.sas.com/en_us/home.html)
MAXQDA (see www.maxqda.com/)	R (see www.r-project.org/)
	Microsoft Excel (see https://products.office.com/en-us/excel)
	Tableau for data visualization (see https://tableau.com)

Summary

In this chapter, we have explored data in rural evaluation contexts. We began this chapter with an overview of typical data sources used in rural evaluation contexts. Then we reviewed these data sources and discussed their quality and use. We ended this chapter with a summary of the different approaches used in analyzing data and the kinds of software available to help us. Evaluators do not have to be statisticians, but they do have to be knowledgeable about the kinds of data they plan to collect, why they are collecting these data, and how they will be analyzed and reported in the evaluation.

Points to remember

1. Data is used to answer evaluation questions.
2. There are various types of data used in rural evaluation contexts. Rural evaluators may collect data with the following considerations in mind: time, location, and population.
3. Data can be collected by rural evaluators, trained community members, and program staff, or it may have been collected by someone else.
4. Always make sure you have appropriate approvals in place before data collection begins. These will vary based on program, community, and funding agency.
5. Evaluation can use qualitative data, quantitative data, or both. Rural evaluators need to be aware of the different data sources available and the approaches used to analyze the data.
6. Various software programs are available to help rural evaluators collect and analyze data. Make sure you are familiar with these programs, their costs, and the skills needed to use these programs before you purchase.

Additional reading and resources

On Reading Levels
How to Assess Reading Level Using Microsoft Word. https://support.office.com/en-us/article/test-your-document-s-readability-85b4969e-e80a-4777-8dd3-f7fc3c8b3fd2

On Probability Sampling and Data Preparation
Trochim, W. (2006). Research Methods Knowledge Base. https://www.socialresearchmethods.net/kb/sampprob.php

On Interviewing
Manzano, A. (2016). The craft of interviewing in realist evaluation. *Evaluation*, *22*(3), 342–360. Retrieved from http://eprints.whiterose.ac.uk/94454/3/Realist Interview-Reviewed.9thOct.pdf

On Focus Groups
Better Evaluation (ND) Conducting Focus Group Interviews. Retrieved from http://www.betterevaluation.org/resources/guides/focus_groups/howto_conduct

On Observation in Evaluation
Richard Krueger (2017). Observation in Evaluation Retrieved from http://www.betterevaluation.org/sites/default/files/Observation%20R.Krueger%2010.17.pdf

On Evaluating Internet Articles
Georgetown University Library (ND). Evaluating Internet Resources. Retrieved from https://www.library.georgetown.edu/tutorials/research-guides/evaluating-internet-content

On Mixed Methods Data Analysis.
Creswell, J. W., & Creswell, J. D. (2017). Research design: Qualitative, quantitative, and mixed methods approaches. Sage publications.

On Statistics
Howell, D. C. (2016). Fundamental statistics for the behavioral sciences. Nelson Education.

On Measurement and Instrumentation
Trochim, W. (2006). Web Center for Social Research Methods. Measurement. Retrieved from http://socialresearchmethods.net/kb/measure.php

On Content Analysis
Hsieh, H. F., & Shannon, S. E. (2005). Three approaches to qualitative content analysis. *Qualitative Health Research, 15*(9), 1277–1288.

On Inductive Approaches
Thomas, D. R. (2006). A general inductive approach for analysing qualitative evaluation data. *American Journal of Evaluation, 27*(2), 237–246.

On Qualitative Methods
Starks, H., & Brown Trinidad, S. (2007). Choose your method: A comparison of phenomenology, discourse analysis, and grounded theory. *Qualitative Health Research*, 17(10), 1372–1380.

Exercises

1. Describe qualitative vs. quantitative data sources used in rural evaluation contexts.
2. List the different kinds of interviews used in evaluation. What are the strengths and limitations of each? Consider rural context and some of the information from Chapters 1–2 in your response.
3. What are some of the questions that you should ask yourself when evaluating Internet articles and data sources in evaluation?

4. What are the primary differences in qualitative and quantitative evaluation approaches?
5. Describe your paradigm as a rural evaluator. How might this influence the data collection and analysis approach you select?
6. Summarize the terms reliability, validity, and content analysis.
7. What are the four primary approaches used in qualitative data analysis? Describe each of these approaches and provide examples of how these approaches can be used in rural evaluation contexts.
8. List some of the software programs used to analyze qualitative and quantitative data. Can you think of others? Find additional software programs not listed, identify the costs of these programs. Does the cost seem reasonable for a rural evaluator or rural program?

Activities

1. Select an evaluation instrument from the Internet, if possible select one that is in MS Word. After you have selected the instrument, assess the readability statistics under the Tools and Options menu in MS Word. What is the readability of the instrument you selected? Do you think it would be appropriate for a rural community member? What if you did not know the literacy level of the population that you were serving? How might you modify your evaluation instrument?
2. Assume you are working in a rural community as an evaluator at a school with 1,000 students. You have been asked to design an evaluation that evaluates student satisfaction with extracurricular activities. Describe the sampling approach you will use. Describe some of the strengths and limitations to using simple random sampling. Are there other sampling approaches that may be more appropriate? Please list and explain your answer.

References

Agency for Toxic Substance Disease Registry15.2 (2015). *Evaluation methods: Community engagement*. Retrieved from https://www.atsdr.cdc.gov/communityengagement/pce_program_methods.html

Attride-Stirling, J. (2001). Thematic networks: An analytic tool for qualitative research. *Qualitative Health Research, 1*, 385–405. doi:10.1177/146879410100100307

Charmaz, K., & McMullen, L. M. (2011). *Five ways of doing qualitative analysis: Phenomenological psychology, grounded theory, discourse analysis, narrative research, and intuitive inquiry*. New York, NY: Guilford Press.

Creswell, J. W., & Creswell, J. D. (2017). *Research design: Qualitative, quantitative, and mixed methods approaches*. Thousand Oaks, CA: Sage Publications.

Creswell, J. W., & Miller, D. L. (2000). Determining validity in qualitative inquiry. *Theory into Practice, 39*(3), 124–130.

Glaser, B. G., & Strauss, A. L. (1967). *The discovery of grounded theory: Strategies for qualitative theory*. New Brunswick, CA: Aldine Transaction.

Golafshani, N. (2003). Understanding reliability and validity in qualitative research. *The Qualitative Report, 8*(4), 597–606.

Good4Utah Local News. *USDA Hosts roundtable focused on the opioid epidemic in rural Utah* April 12, 2018 by Jen Jacobson. Retrieved from http://www.good4utah.com/news/local-news/roundtable-focuses-on-opioid-epidemic-in-utah/1117341054

Guba, E. G., & Lincoln, Y. S. (1989). *Fourth generation evaluation.* Newbury Park, CA: Sage Publications.

Gubrium, A., & Turner, K. N. (2011). Digital storytelling as an emergent method for social research and practice. In S. N. Hesse-Biber (Ed.), *The handbook of emergent technologies in social research* (pp. 469–491). New York, NY: Oxford University Press.

Guest, G., Bunce, A., & Johnson, L. (2006). How many interviews are enough? An experiment with data saturation and variability. *Field Methods, 18,* 59–82.

Hernon, P., & Schwartz, C. (2009). *Quantitative research: Reliability and validity. Student affairs assessment, Portland State University.* Retrieved from https://www.pdx.edu/studentaffairs/sites/www.pdx.edu.studentaffairs/files/QuanRshRel&Val.pdf

Hsieh, H. F., & Shannon, S. E. (2005). Three approaches to qualitative content analysis. *Qualitative Health Research, 15*(9), 1277–1288.

Johnson, R. B., Onwuegbuzie, A. J., & Turner, L. A. (2007). Toward a definition of mixed methods research. *Journal of Mixed Methods Research, 1*(2), 112–133.

Kahn, J. (2010). *Reporting statistics in APA Style.* Illinois State University. Retrieved from http://my.ilstu.edu/~jhkahn/apastats.html

Kelley, A., Medicine Bull, K., & LaFranier, G. (2016). Participatory visual methods for American Indian communities and mental health conversations. *American Indian and Alaska Native Mental Health Research* (Online), *23*(1), 47.

Krueger, R. (2017). *Observation in Evaluation. University of Minnesota.* Retrieved from http://www.betterevaluation.org/sites/default/files/Observation%20R.Krueger%2010.17.pdf

Lasch, K. E., Marquis, P., Vigneux, M., Abetz, L., Arnould, B., & Bayliss, M. (2010). PRO development: Rigorous qualitative research as the crucial foundation. *Quality of Life Research, 19*(8), 1087–1096. doi:10.1007/s11136-010-9677-6

Manzano, A. (2016). The craft of interviewing in realist evaluation. *Evaluation, 22*(3), 342–360.

Mertens, D. M. (2014). *Research and evaluation in education and psychology: Integrating diversity with quantitative, qualitative, and mixed methods.* Thousand Oaks, CA: Sage Publications.

Monette, D. R., Sullivan, T. J., & DeJong, C. R. (1990). *Applied social research: Tool for the human services* (p. 337). Fort Worth, TX: Holt, Rinehart and Winston.

Rice, W. R. (1989). Analyzing tables of statistical tests. *Evolution, 43*(1), 223–225.

Rose, S., Spinks, N., & Canhoto, A. I. (2015). *Tests for the assumption that a variable is normally distributed. Management research: Applying the principles.* Retrieved from http://documents.routledge-interactive.s3.amazonaws.com/9780415628129/Chapter%209%20-%20Determining%20sample%20size%20final_edited.pdf

Rumsey, D. J., & Unger, D. (2015). *U can: Statistics for dummies.* New York, NY. John Wiley & Sons.

Schwandt, T. A. (2001). *Dictionary of qualitative inquiry,* 2nd edition. Thousand Oaks, CA: Sage Publications.

Simpson, S. H. (2015). Creating a data analysis plan: What to consider when choosing statistics for a study. *The Canadian Journal of Hospital Pharmacy, 68*(4), 311–317.

Starks, H., & Trinidad, S. B. (2007). Choose your method: A comparison of phenomenology, discourse analysis, and grounded theory. *Qualitative Health Research, 17*(10), 1372–1380.

Taylor-Powell, E. (1998). Collecting group data: Nominal group technique, Quick tips. In *Program development and evaluation* (pp. 1–12). Madison, WI: University of Wisconsin-Extension, Cooperative Extension.

Thomas, D. R. (2006). A general inductive approach for analysing qualitative evaluation data. *American Journal of Evaluation, 27*(2), 237–246.

Trochim, W. (2006). *Web center for research methods knowledge base.* Retrieved from https://www.socialresearchmethods.net/kb/sampprob.php

Web Center for Social Research Methods (2006). *Probability sampling.* Retrieved from https://www.socialresearchmethods.net/kb/sampprob.php

Wilcox, S., Castro, C., King, A. C., Houseman, R., & Brownson, R. (2000). Determinants of leisure time physical activity in rural compared with urban older and ethnically diverse women in the United States. *Journal of Epidemiology & Community Health, 54,* 667–672. doi:10.1136/jech.54.9.667

Wodak, R., & Meyer, M. (Eds.). (2009). *Methods for critical discourse analysis.* London: Sage Publications.

7

DOCUMENTING THE PROCESS, OUTCOME/IMPACT, AND ECONOMIC PROGRAM EVALUATION

For the longest time I knew what evaluation was, I understood the terms, but I did not know how to document evaluation. I searched for examples, but I found few. This was one of the biggest challenges that I experienced early in my career. This chapter might seem redundant, but it is for you to read, take, and use. It is my sincere hope that through this chapter you will learn how to document evaluation in a way that resonates with you and the community you serve.

Program evaluation started in the 1800s when the federal government called for inspectors to evaluate public programs, schools, and hospitals (Stufflebeam, Madaus, & Kellaghan, 2000). Evaluation continued to evolve through the 1930s when social systems were rapidly changing, then in the 1960s, the Great Society Legislation was passed and this legislation required program evaluation. The Great Society Legislation was designed to eliminate poverty and racial injustice, and several programs were developed to address education, medical care, rural poverty, and transportation needs. Today nearly every discipline utilizes evaluation and evaluators represent diverse backgrounds in education, psychology, statistics, and other social science fields.

In this chapter, we will highlight the purpose, questions, and timing for different program evaluation approaches. Each section will end with an example to extend our thinking about documenting evaluation results and dissemination.

Formative evaluation

Purpose. Documenting formative evaluation in rural communities focuses on accountability, monitoring resource use, and documenting progress and challenges that may occur. **Questions**. Have activities been conducted as planned? Have services been offered as a result of the program? Has the effort accomplished what it intended? **Timing**. May occur when a new program is developed, when a program has been modified, or as needed. **Case example**. The "Formative evaluation for a healthy corner store initiative in Pitt County, North Carolina", is an example of how a formative evaluation was designed, documented, and disseminated (Box 7.1).

BOX 7.1 Formative evaluation of the healthy corner store initiative

Formative evaluation for a healthy corner store initiative in Pitt County, North Carolina: Assessing the rural food environment, Part 1 (Jilcott et al., 2013)

Introduction: Obesity disparities in rural areas may be the result of the food environment and rural food deserts. Previous research indicates that rural residents may depend more on corner stores (convenience stores or food marts) than their urban counterparts. Because rural residents live farther from supermarkets than their urban- and suburban-dwelling counterparts, they may be more reliant on smaller corner stores that offer fewer healthful food items.

Federal support: The Centers for Disease Control and Prevention Communities Putting Prevention to Work initiative included $372.9 million to plan and evaluate healthful food initiatives in rural communities throughout America.

Evaluation methods: Evaluators reviewed audit tools in the fall of 2010 to measure the consumer food environment in eastern North Carolina and chose the NEMS-S-Rev (Nutrition Environment Measures Survey-Stores-Revised) to assess 42 food stores.

Data collection: During the spring and summer of 2011, two trained graduate assistants audited stores, achieving interrater reliability of at least 80%. NEMS-S-Rev scores of stores in rural versus urban areas were compared.

Results: Overall, healthful foods were less available and of lower quality in rural areas than in urban areas.

Conclusion: Food store audit data provided a baseline to implement and evaluate the Centers for Disease Control and Prevention Communities Putting Prevention to Work (CPPW) healthy corner store initiative in Pitt County. This work serves as a case study, providing lessons learned for engaging community partners when conducting rural food store audits.

Dissemination: Evaluators published the results of this formative evaluation in a peer reviewed journal, *Preventing Chronic Disease*. The results were also shared with community members, policy makers, and corner store owners. The goal of dissemination was to promote more healthful food choices in rural and underserve areas while advocating for policy and environmental changes in the rural America.

Source: Jilcott Pitts et al. (2013)

Process evaluation

Purpose. Documenting the process evaluation provides critical information for making program modifications. **Questions.** Is the program being implemented as planned and on schedule? What are the strengths and weaknesses? **Timing.** Begins when an evaluation plan is developed (see Chapter 5), at the beginning of a program and during implementation. **Case example.** Process evaluation of a promotora de salud intervention for improving hypertension outcomes for Latinos living in a rural US–Mexico border region (Box 7.2).

BOX 7.2 Process evaluation of a promotora de salud intervention

Background: Rates of hypertension among US–Mexico border Latinos is a growing public health problem due to limited awareness and lack of treatment and control options. Authors developed a nine-week promotora de salud-led curriculum in two rural communities located in the New Mexico. The curriculum helps facilitate participant's engagement in managing hypertension.

Theoretical foundation: Social support and social cognitive theories.

Evaluation method: Process evaluation to assess Corazon po la Vida curriculum delivery.

Evaluation questions: Were the sessions implemented as designed? Was the curriculum fully implemented? What was the quality of delivery? How many sessions did participants complete?

Evaluation measures: Process evaluation measures included adherence, quality of delivery, participant responsiveness, and dosage. Participant measures included self-reported diet and physical activity information. An assessment of community resources was also used because they support chronic disease management.

Data collection: Response data was collected at three different time points from 260 participants.

Data analysis: Descriptive statistics, factor analysis, correlation matrix.

Results: Ninety-six Latino participants completed at least one session. Promotora reported teaching 100% of the content for 95 of the 99 sessions. Promotoras reported that 81% of the participants were satisfied with the sessions. Attendance was 77.47% for education sessions. Higher doses of the intervention were associated with improved self-reported outcomes. Community resources to support improved health behaviors did not have any significant effect for participants.

Changes made during the intervention: Promotoras made changes to improve the uptake of information, and make it more culturally responsive and age appropriate. Promotoras changed the session order, combined and modified materials, and changed and omitted some activities. As participation (dose) in the program increased, self-reported health outcomes improved.

Dissemination: Results were published in the journal, *Health Promotion Practice*. Authors also advocated for a national research agenda that ensures effective interventions for Latino populations. This was one of the first evaluations to document an effective public health intervention for rural/frontier Latino populations in the United States. Promotoras are effective and should be integrated into health teams in rural and frontier communities throughout America.

Source: Sánchez et al. (2014)

Outcome evaluation

Purpose. Outcome evaluations are used to document if the desired outcomes were achieved and what made a program effective or ineffective. Outcome evaluations also explore the likelihood that a program can be sustained or replicated. **Questions.** What changes did the program cause? How did the program contribute to these changes? How is the effort going to be sustained and replicated? **Timing.** After program implementation begins or when program is stable. **Case example.** The evaluation "Evaluating early numeracy skills in preschool children: A program evaluation of rural head start classrooms" is one example of an outcome evaluation (Box 7.3).

BOX 7.3 Outcome evaluation of rural head start classrooms

Evaluating early numeracy skills in preschool children: A program evaluation of rural head start classrooms (Alger, 2015)

Background: Early numeracy skills are a critical component of daily preschool instruction, according to the National Council of Teachers of Mathematics. However, there is variability in how mathematics-driven instruction is delivered. This evaluation focused on selected mathematics curriculum utilized by a head start program.

Participants: Participants were children enrolled in the head start classes in a rural, western New York State county, and their classroom teachers. Within the organization, there are a total of 10 Head Start class-rooms with approximately 20 students in six communities serving 200 children annually.

Evaluator: The evaluator was a doctoral student at Alfred University in the School of Psychology, College of Professional Studies, Division of Counseling and School Psychology. This evaluation was her dissertation. The author's connection to rural head start classrooms and the target population is not clear.

Evaluation design: Five of the ten classrooms were randomly selected for inclusion in the experimental group; the remaining five classrooms were assigned to the control group. One hundred students were initially included in the experimental group and approximately 100 students in the control group. Approximately 10 teachers were included in the study, with five randomly assigned to the experimental group that implemented the new curriculum, and the remaining five assigned to the control group.

Data analysis: The evaluator analyzed demographic data from students and teachers. Correlations were used to explore relationships between the two math measures of interests. The evaluator also used independent samples t-tests and Chi-square goodness-of-fit tests to document statistical differences between the control and experimental groups. Sequential multiple regression models were used to explore student and teacher variables on the mathematics outcome scores as measured by the posttest scores. Other data from the Weekly Math Logs were analyzed qualitatively.

Findings: The results indicated that children's mathematics achievement was below established targets. The results also indicated that the curriculum did not show significant gains in math skills compared to children in the control group.

Dissemination: The evaluator published these results in her dissertation (June 2015). Other dissemination efforts are not known.

Source: Alger (2015)

Impact evaluation

Purpose. Impact evaluations review positive and negative program effects, determine if effects are intended or unintended, help establish accountability, and contribute to lessons learned. Impact evaluation requires counterfactual evidence of what outcomes would be without a program. **Questions.** What is the overall impact of the program? What is the nature of impacts and their reach? What influence did other factors have on the impacts? How did the program contribute to impacts? Are impacts sustainable? How? Did the impacts match the needs of the target population? What would have happened without the

program? **Timing.** After the program has been implemented and there is suf-
ficient data to answer impact questions and document impact. **Case example.**
Impact Evaluation of the US Department of Education's Student Mentoring
Program (Box 7.4).

BOX 7.4 Impact evaluation of the US Department of Education

Program: The US Department of Education's Student Mentoring Program
is a competitive federal grant program managed by the Office of Safe and
Drug-Free Schools in both rural and urban communities throughout America. The program addresses the lack of supportive adults in at-risk students
by funding schools and community using faith-based organizations targeting
children in grades 4–8.

Evaluator: The Institute of Education Sciences (IES) National Center
for Education Evaluation and Regional Assistance oversaw the independent
evaluation. Abt Associates and a team of subcontractors, Branch Associates,
Moore and Associates, and the Center for Resource Management, worked as
a team to conduct the evaluation.

Evaluation design: A student-level random assignment design focusing
on the impacts of the Student Mentoring Program on students randomly
assigned to participate in the US Department of Education (ED) mentoring
programs compared to similar students who signed up to participate, but
were not assigned to participate in the programs.

Selection: Thirty-two purposively selected School Mentoring Programs
and 2,573 students took part in the evaluation.

Evaluation questions: What is the impact of ED school-based mentoring programs on students' interpersonal relationships with adults, personal
responsibility, and community involvement? What is the impact of ED school-
based mentoring programs on students' school engagement and academic
achievement? What is the impact of ED school-based mentoring programs
on students' high-risk or delinquent behavior?

Outcome measures: The evaluation team reviewed 17 outcomes in the
domains of interpersonal relationships and personal responsibility, academic
achievement and engagement, and high-risk or delinquent behavior.

Analytic approach: The evaluation team used a fixed-effects model to
estimate the average treatment effect across all programs for students assigned to receive mentoring versus students assigned to an untreated control
group.

Impacts: A total of 17 impacts in three domains: (1) academic achievement and engagement, (2) interpersonal relationships and personal responsibility, and (3) high-risk or delinquent behavior were noted.

Results: The impact evaluation of the Student Mentoring Program did not lead to statistically significant impacts on students in any of the three outcome domains. The Student Mentoring Program led to a decrease in truancy for younger students.

Dissemination: This report was summarized and posted on the Institute of Educational Sciences (IES) National Center for Education Evaluation (NCEE) website. Other dissemination mediums may have been used, but they are not articulated in the report.

Source: US Department of Education (2009)

Assessment

Purpose. Assessments are used to monitor and document how programs are being implemented and the changes that need to be made. Rural evaluators use various types of assessments, and needs assessments are one example. **Questions**. What is known? What is needed? What has changed? What needs to change? **Timing**. Can be used before and after a program, to make changes, or to inform program strategy and direction. Use of assessment is to monitor how the program is being implemented and make changes to improve process and outcomes. **Case example**. Listening to rural Hispanic immigrants in the Midwest: a community-based participatory assessment of major barriers to health care access and use (Box 7.5).

BOX 7.5 Participatory assessment of barriers to health care

Program: This impact evaluation assessment is part of a Hispanic community health needs assessment effort. Project Excellence in Partnerships for Community Outreach, Research and Training (EXPORT) focuses on reducing health disparities among racial and ethnic groups in rural underserved populations in Illinois. In the last 10 years, 14 communities served by EXPORT have witnessed a 263% increase in Hispanic growth.

Assessment team: Project EXPORT includes a community outreach team that works in partnership with local advisory committees.

Selection: Participants were three rural communities in Illinois. To be included in the assessment communities had to be involved in Project EXPORT activities, have a local Hispanic advisory committee, be in a nonmetropolitan area, and have significant growth of at least 30% Hispanic residents between 1990 and 2000. Focus group participants were recruited by advisory council members using promotional flyers written in Spanish, and posted at Mexican grocery stores, restaurants, community centers, libraries, and churches.

Consent: Because of differences in literacy levels, participants gave verbal consent and received a paper copy of the consent form.

Design: The Project EXPORT assessment team worked with local Hispanic advisory councils to plan and design focused small group discussions to document the main barriers that participants experience when accessing and utilizing health care services. The design was based on qualitative data, community-based participatory research methods, and participatory action research methods.

Groups: Focused group discussions lasted between 60 and 90 minutes.

Analysis: Moderators and assistants transcribed notes from group discussion and then translated them into English. Data were analyzed independently by two bilingual coders and then compared across categories.

Results: Themes resulting from the focused groups and analyses indicate that the main barriers encountered when accessing health care services include lack of health insurance, high cost, communication issues, legal status and lack of documentation, discrimination, and transportation issues.

Limitations: Findings are not generalizable to other rural Hispanic population in the United States. Rural Hispanics from other regions in the United States may be from Central or South America and have different issues than the population involved in this assessment.

Dissemination: Peer-reviewed journal article.

Source: Cristancho, Peters and Muller (2008)

Economic evaluation

Purpose. Economic evaluations are conducted to document the costs of a program, to reduce program costs, and to monitor program effectiveness. The results from economic evaluations are used to inform and influence policy, and support informed decision-making. **Questions.** What are the total program costs? What are the cost savings that resulted from the program (health, environment, human life, other)? What is the net cost? **Timing.** At the beginning of a program, during a program, or after a program has been implemented. There must be sufficient cost and outcome data to document cost savings from program delivery. **Case example**. Kentucky Homeplace program (Box 7.6).

Here is another example: "A cost–benefit analysis of physical activity using bike/pedestrian trails" (Wang et al., 2005) (Box 7.7).

BOX 7.6 Economic evaluation of Kentucky Homeplace program

Background: Kentucky Homeplace was founded in 1994 by the University of Kentucky Center for Excellence in Rural Health. Kentucky Homeplace serves 30 counties in the Appalachian region of eastern Kentucky. Most residents experience poverty, unemployment, lower educational attainment, inadequate health insurance, and transportation barriers.

Program services: Kentucky Homeplace trains community health workers to provide access to health and social services. Community health workers are members of the community, born and raised in rural Appalachia. Services include a variety of preventive health services, eye exams and glasses, hearing aids, reduced and no-cost medications, reduced and low-cost dental services, referral visits, enrolment, in Medicaid and children's health insurance, and Medicare part D.

Enumerating costs: Authors reviewed client data from July 2001 to June 2016 from 152,262 Kentucky Homeplace clients. Kentucky Homeplace provided 4,748,727 services with a service value of $308,335,241. The return on investment was $11.55 saved for every $1 spent. Note that the length of time under review (15 years) allows for sufficient cost and outcome data to document cost savings.

Dissemination: Quarterly Reports, peer reviewed publications, model has been recognized by state, local, and federal policy makers for supporting policy and systems change, and expanding community health worker roles in the health care delivery system.

Source: Rural Health Information Hub (2018)

BOX 7.7 Cost–benefit of bike/pedestrian trails

Background: Physical inactivity is a risk factor for a variety of chronic diseases. To document and maintain the cost benefits of physical activity using bike and pedestrian trails in Lincoln, Nebraska, economists from the Centers for Disease Control designed the study entitled "A cost–benefit analysis of physical activity using bike/pedestrian trails" (Wang et al., 2005).

Data and methods used: Wang and colleagues reviewed existing data from the Lincoln Recreational Trails Census Report 1998, and agency correspondence (2005). Other data included information about the trails, how long they were, when they were built, and the kinds of materials used to construct them.

Enumerating costs: Authors determined that trails could be used for an average of 30 years and costs associated with construction and maintenance were adjusted to 1998 dollars (to match the year of the Census Report). Trail use and costs were calculated by dividing the total trail costs by the number of trail uses per year. Equipment and travel were estimated at $100 per year based on previous research. Health benefits from physical activity and trail use were measured using the difference in direct medical costs for active persons compared with inactive persons.

Cost–benefit ratio: Wang and colleagues developed a cost–benefit ratio by totaling the direct medical cost savings and dividing this by the total trail costs (construction, maintenance, equipment, and travel). A cost–benefit ratio greater than one indicates that positive benefit and positive return on funds invested. A cost–benefit ratio less than one indicates that there were more funds invested than returned (in savings or benefit).

Results: According to this study, the cost to build a trail averaged $1.35 million, the annual average cost was $44,949, and trail maintenance averaged $15,445 per year. Trails were used an average of 225,351 times and the average cost per use was $0.27. Costs for trail users were calculated at 52 weeks, three times per week, and $0.27 per use, thus $52 \times 3 \times \$0.27 = \$42.12$. Wang and colleagues then included $150 for equipment and travel, increasing the total annual costs per trail to $192.12 ($42.12 + $150) (2005). Want reported the direct health benefit for individuals using the trail as $564.41. This number or benefit was then divided by the total costs per trail user, $192.12. The cost–benefit ratio (CBR) was $564.41/$192.12=2.94. A CBR of 2.94 means that, for every $1 invested, there was a direct medical benefit of $2.94.

Dissemination: The results were published in an academic journal, *Health Promotion and Practice*. Since authors were employed at the Centers for Disease Control, it is likely that these results were used to promote physical activity through various prevention task forces at the Centers for Disease Control. Economic benefits and results from this study were also posted on the American Trails website: www.americantrails.org/resources/economics/economic-benefits-trails-macdonald.html and the Headwaters Economics website: https://headwaterseconomics.org/trail/93-ne-cost-benefit-analysis-physical-activity/.

Source: Wang et al. (2005)

Summary

In this chapter, we reinforced our knowledge of formative, process, assessment, outcome, impact, and economic evaluations using case examples from rural America. In some case examples, it was not clear what type of evaluation was being used, and in other cases, authors used the type of evaluation in the title. As a rural evaluator, it is important to be clear about the evaluation approach used, the purpose, questions, and timing—doing this will help ensure that evaluation results are used as intended. There are several important lessons from this chapter. Evaluation takes time and skills. Evaluation also has a purpose and must be flexible and tailored to fit the community and program needs—as a rural evaluator, you can make this happen.

Points to remember

1. There are various types of evaluation that rural evaluators use. Select a type that is most appropriate for the community, context, and purpose.
2. Process evaluation is useful for documenting what is working, why it works, if the program has been implemented as planned, and what needs to be improved.
3. Outcome evaluation is used when we want to know what changes the program caused and how the program contributed to these challenges.
4. Impact evaluation helps us determine the overall impact of a program, the nature of these impacts, and their reach. Impact evaluation also helps us to document impacts and which impacts are sustainable overtime.
5. Economic evaluation focuses on the cost of the program and the savings that resulted from the program.
6. Be flexible. Make sure the evaluation fits the needs of the community and fulfills the program purpose.

Additional reading and resources

On Outcome Evaluation
Kay Rockwell & Claude Bennett (2004). Targeting Outcomes of Programs: A Hierarchy for Targeting Outcomes and Evaluating Their Achievement. Faculty Publications: Agricultural, Leadership, Education & Communication Department. Paper 48. Retrieved from http://www.meera.snre.umich.edu/sites/all/files/Rockwell%20and%20Bennett.pdf

On Impact Evaluation
Patricia Rogers (2012). An Introduction to Impact Evaluation. RMIT University Australia and Better Evaluation.

On Selecting High Performance Indicators
Goldie MacDonald (ND). A Checklist to Inform Monitoring and Evaluation. Centres for Disease Control Retrieved from https://www.wmich.edu/sites/default/files/attachments/u350/2014/Indicator_checklist.pdf

On Program Evaluation
Kellogg Foundation (2010). W.K. Kellogg Foundation Evaluation Handbook. Retrieved from https://www.wkkf.org/resource-directory/resource/2010/w-k-kellogg-foundation-evaluation-handbook

On Economic Evaluation
Centers for Disease Control and Prevention (2018). Five Part Webcast on Economic Evaluation. Retrieved from https://www.cdc.gov/dhdsp/evaluation_resources/economic_evaluation/index.htm

Chapter questions

1. Describe the purpose of process, outcome, impact, assessment, and economic evaluation. What are the similarities? What are the differences? How might these approaches be challenged by rural context and limited resources?
2. How is the timing of each evaluation approach different? What do rural evaluators need to remember about timing the evaluation?
3. What are the differences in evaluation examples that use qualitative data, quantitative data, or both? What are some of the strengths and weaknesses of using qualitative, quantitative, or both in rural communities?
4. Which case example(s) mentioned a theory? For the case examples that did not mention a theory, can you identify a theory that might have been used in planning the evaluation?
5. Summarize the main points of the economic evaluation case examples in this chapter. When is economic evaluation feasible in rural community evaluation? What are the challenges of economic evaluation in rural communities and how might you overcome these?
6. Review the assessment case example. List one example of how rural evaluators might use assessment in their work.

Activities

1. Use the Internet and search the terms "Impact Evaluation Rural United States". Select one of the results. Review the impact evaluation. Who was the author? Describe the program/intervention being evaluated? What study design did they use? What were the limitations of the impact evaluation? How were results disseminated? Is there evidence of policy change, advocacy, or reform as a result of the evaluation?

References

Alger, M. (2015). *Evaluating early numeracy skills in preschool children: A program evaluation of rural head start classrooms.* Dissertation. College of Professional Studies, Alfred University. Retrieved from https://aura.alfred.edu/bitstream/handle/10829/6941/Alger%2c%20Megan%202015.pdf?sequence=1&isAllowed=y

Cristancho, S., Garces, D. M., Peters, K. E., & Mueller, B. C. (2008). Listening to rural hispanic immigrants in the Midwest: A community-based participatory assessment of major barriers to health care access and use. *Qualitative Health Research, 18*(5), 633–646.

Pitts, S. B. J., Bringolf, K. R., Lloyd, C. L., McGuirt, J. T., Lawton, K. K., & Morgan, J. (2013). Peer reviewed: Formative evaluation for a healthy corner store initiative in pitt county, North Carolina: Engaging stakeholders for a healthy corner store initiative, part 2. *Preventing chronic disease*, 10: E120. Retrieved from: https://www.ncbi.nlm.nih.gov/pmc/articles/PMC3716339/

Rural Health Information Hub (2018). *Case Studies and Conversations, Models and Innovations. Kentucky Homeplace Program.* Retrieved from https://www.ruralhealthinfo.org/project-examples/785

Sánchez, V., Cacari Stone, L., Moffett, M. L., Nguyen, P., Muhammad, M., Bruna-Lewis, S., & Urias-Chauvin, R. (2014). Process evaluation of a promotora de salud intervention for improving hypertension outcomes for Latinos living in a rural US–Mexico border region. *Health Promotion Practice, 15*(3), 356–364.

Stufflebeam, D. L., Madaus, G. F., & Kellaghan, T. (Eds.). (2000). *Evaluation models: Viewpoints on educational and human services evaluation* (Vol. 49). New York, NY: Springer Science & Business Media.

U.S. Department of Education (2009). *Impact Evaluation of the U.S. Department of Education's Student Mentoring Program. Final Report NCEE 2009–4047.* Retrieved from https://permanent.access.gpo.gov/LPS117460/LPS117460/ies.ed.gov/ncee/pubs/20094047/pdf/20094047.pdf

Wang, G., Macera, C. A., Scudder-Soucie, B., Schmid, T., Pratt, M., & Buchner, D. (2005). A cost-benefit analysis of physical activity using bike/pedestrian trails. *Health Promotion Practice, 6*, 174–179.

8

REPORTING AND APPLICATION OF RURAL EVALUATION FINDINGS

What I have learned about reporting results and applying findings in rural evaluation has taken some time. Early in my work I thought that everyone would want to know and read everything. I developed long evaluation reports with citations and support from academic journals. But the people who would benefit from reading the reports never actually read them. Now, I know there are different approaches in reporting. Short reports, infographics, and summaries are some of the best ways to highlight evaluation results and apply them to create action steps for change and program improvement. Comprehensive evaluation reports include everything—they are important because they serve as a track record for what you did, what the program did, how it was evaluated, and what it meant.

Once you have collected the evaluation data, analyzed the data, and written up the results, it is time to report the evaluation findings to stakeholders, policy makers, community stakeholders, and the funding agency. When reporting evaluation findings in rural communities, always be aware of the context, how people get information, when they get it, how they might use it, and why it is important.

Reporting evaluation findings

When reporting the evaluation findings, consider this five-step process (Figure 8.1)

Engage

Stakeholders are individuals who are engaged, supportive, and involved in a program and evaluation. Stakeholders can help plan how evaluation findings will be applied and disseminated during the early stages of evaluation planning.

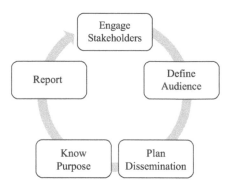

FIGURE 8.1   Five-Step Process for Reporting Evaluation Results.

Stakeholders can also help review evaluation findings and add contextual information that helps clarify and validate results, along with developing recommendations for future action and work (CDC, 2013). To ensure that stakeholders are engaged in the evaluation planning and dissemination process, it is important to have a relationship with them, and to know the best ways to communicate with them.

Define

Define the target audience or recipients of the evaluation findings. Different audiences need to know different information that is presented in different ways. Consider a 400-page evaluation report that is submitted to a funding agency at the end of a program. This lengthy report is likely too long for policy makers who have limited time and want to know the main actions or recommendations from an evaluation. A verbal presentation with a short five-page summary that highlights the evaluation approach, findings, and recommendations may be more appropriate for policy makers. When considering the target audience, consider the community, context, literacy levels, and information that are most salient to the goals of the program and community. The Centers for Disease Control and Prevention recommends seven things to keep in mind when defining your target audience: have effective communication challenges, determine what action should be taken, know the technical expertise and comprehension level of your audience, make sure the information is culturally responsive, know the expectations of the audience, present information based on what is most appropriate for the community, and consider how the audience may interpret findings (CDC, 2013).

Plan

Develop a dissemination plan that targets your intended audiences and the information they need to know, in a manner that is consistent with community expectations, norms, and culture. Dissemination plans generally define the target audience, the medium that will be used to share results, when findings will be used, the person responsible, resources available, follow-up actions, and monitoring follow-up activities.

Be clear and know the purpose

Know the purpose of the evaluation and what the community expects to see in the evaluation report. Evaluations have several purposes. Some evaluations are used to gain insight and understanding about a new program or intervention. Others are used to improve programs and practices. Evaluations can be used to document the relationship between programs and interventions and outcomes, or to determine their value.

The evaluation report

Determine the type of evaluation report that will be used to share results. Traditional evaluation reports serve four main purposes: (1) add knowledge and understanding about the program and evaluation practice, (2) provide context about the community or setting along with any relevant background information, (3) create a basis for other reports and communications, and (4) establish accountability. Consider written, verbal, and electronic reports—make sure these reports are action oriented and focus on findings and next steps (CDC, 2013).

Presenting data

Evaluation reports, presentations, and communications will include data, often qualitative and quantitative. Stephanie Evergreen's book, *Presenting Data Effectively*, is a must read for evaluators who are using data to communicate results of a program evaluation. The uptake of information from an evaluation report occurs in three distinct phases: early attention, working memory, and long-term memory (Evergreen, 2017). When developing an evaluation report, use images, photographs, and graphs to help readers understand information presented and retain the information for future use (Evergreen, 2017). Use data formats that are familiar to the target audience and explain the data when appropriate (Nelson, Hesse, & Croyle, 2009). Basic design principles should be followed when presenting data, and these principles include appropriate use of graphics, color, typeface, and organization. Graphics include photographs, figures, and images. Effective graphics should be emotional, placed for high impact, communicate with intention, and repeated (Evergreen, 2017). Typeface or fonts help us communicate results more clearly and effectively. Typically text fonts are used in narrative text and the size of the font ranges from 9- to 11-point size. Heading type face should be 150%–200% of the narrative text size. If you are using an

11-point font size for your narrative, the heading font size would need to be between 16- and 22-point size. Line spacing is typically 11–13 points. Headings, subheadings, narrative text, captions, and callouts emphasize key points. Colors in reports help readers remember and focus on specific information. Determine what kind of report you will be developing; printed evaluation reports use Red Blue Green color codes, while electronic or screen viewed evaluation reports use Cyan, magenta, yellow, and key black color. When selecting a color for the background and the font, the most important thing to keep in mind is the contrast between the two colors. Typically, margins are set at 1-inch on the top, bottom, and each side. Make sure that the line length of the report is between 8 and 12 words per line. If you are using graphics, images, or tables, make sure that you support these with text. If you have placed a pie chart on a page without any narrative, the reader might be drawn to the pie chart, but not fully understand what it means or how it links to the evaluation findings. Last, make sure you arrange information in a logical way, where the most salient information in your evaluation report takes up the most space and is in the front of the report.

There are various software programs available for creating reports, ranging from Adobe InDesign, Lucid Press, and Pictochart to Microsoft Word or Publisher. Review these programs and select the one that is right for you and the community you serve.

Basic elements of an evaluation report

Executive summary

The executive summary is a brief narrative that highlights the evaluation results. Typically, this is just one page and gives the reader enough information to know the background, purpose, methods, findings, recommendations, and lessons learned (Box 8.1).

BOX 8.1 Field notes on an executive summary

Background: The report summarizes findings from a process and outcome evaluation. The findings are based on three leadership activities and one focus group that occurred in a rural community during a three-week period in 2018. Leadership activities were facilitated by a youth development specialist and facilitating program staff at a local school. A focus group explored youth perceptions of leadership opportunities in the area and identified the ways in which they engage in leadership activities.

Purpose and method: This mixed-methods evaluation was grounded in youth leadership theory. A doctoral trained evaluator facilitated the data analyses process using MS Excel, SPSS version 24.0, and NVivo version 11.0. Primary data sources used in this study were: field notes, email communications, observation, activity evaluations, focus group transcripts, youth leadership survey results, youth quality of life survey results, and photographs from various leadership activities. Data sources were triangulated to answer the primary research question, "What are the best ways to engage youth in leadership activities in this rural community?".

Findings: Results from the evaluation underscore the need for opportunities that allow youth to engage in leadership activities and develop prosocial relationships with their peers. We learned that youth most often access leadership activities through school-based clubs. The best ways to engage youth in leadership activities is to partner with existing community programs, schools, and services. Our youth participants felt that family services, churches, schools, and local gyms like the YMCA would be good partners for future efforts.

Recommendations: We encountered five primary challenges in the implementation of this leadership program that are explored in detail: initial focus on youth stress was not appropriate for the population and the leadership activities planned, transportation and scheduling, recruitment and retention, and multiple project leads.

Discussion and implications: This was the first evaluation that explored youth leadership development within the context of youth living in the community. This was also the first program initiated by the school to explore youth leadership needs. The results underscore the need for continued efforts that give youth the opportunity to develop their leadership skills and improve their quality of life.

Background

Historical information about a community, program, or intervention is important because it provides context and helps the reader get familiar with a program, a need, and the evaluation purpose. The background information should include a statement of need. Often the statement of need is described using baseline statistics that document need for the program or intervention. Often the background section includes a statement on the organization facilitating the program, their mission, vision, and goals and how the program or intervention fits within the organization's mission.

Evaluation purpose

Clearly define the evaluation with a purpose statement. Purpose statements include the reason for the evaluation and how the findings will be used. Due to the

---

BOX 8.2 Field notes on evaluation purpose

The purpose of this evaluation is to document the best ways to engage youth in leadership activities. The results obtained from the evaluation will be documented in a report and shared with school administrators, the funding agency, participants, and community stakeholders.

---

nature of rural communities, sometimes the purpose and reasons change. In rural communities, there may be changes in who the stakeholders are, new community leaders may be elected or identified, and the need for the evaluation and the results may change as a result of new programming, policy, or funding—revisit these areas to ensure utility of evaluation. Program and organizational changes are also important to revisit because they can directly impact how the evaluation results will be used (CDC, 2013) (see Box 8.2).

Methods

The methods section of your evaluation report should include five components: design, data, target population, analysis, and limitations. Using your evaluation plan and data collection strategy, documents will be helpful when writing the methods section of your report (Box 8.3).

BOX 8.3 Field notes on evaluation methods

Design: We used a mixed-methods evaluation design to answer the primary evaluation question, "What are the best ways to engage youth in leadership activities in this rural community?".

Data: Primary data sources used in this study were: field notes, email communications, observation, activity evaluations, focus group transcripts, youth leadership survey results, youth quality of life survey results, and photographs from various leadership activities. Data were triangulated to gain a more comprehensive understanding of youth leadership opportunities, focus areas, and partnerships for future work.

Target population: Our target population was youth between the ages of 13–18 years. Youth had to be in grades 7–12 at the time of recruitment and understand spoken and written English. We recruited youth from middle and high schools from the rural community beginning in September 2017.

Analysis: We analyzed quantitative data from the youth leadership survey and youth quality of life survey using MS Excel and SPSS version 24.0.

Qualitative data from open text responses and focus groups were transcribed and analyzed using NVIVO Software version 11.0. Photographs, study team meeting minutes and notes, and statements from youth and program staff were uploaded into a shared file to contextualize responses.

Limitations: We explored leadership within the context of a rural Oregon community using a small sample of youth—this limits the generalizability and application of our findings, but does not diminish their importance. Second, youth participants did not share a lot of information during the focus groups and this limited the amount of qualitative data available to answer our primary evaluation question.

Key findings

This section highlights the most important results from the evaluation. When writing your key findings, make sure that you use language that is easy to understand. Consider using photographs, tables, figures, bullets, and headers to emphasize areas that you want the audience to read (Box 8.4).

BOX 8.4 Field notes on key findings

Key findings that emerged from the evaluation of this leadership program may be useful as the school moves forward with youth leadership development efforts.

The program documented the need for leadership activities that reach rural youth. Youth participants did not feel that there were a lot of opportunities for leadership development in their community.

School program staff may consider exploring outdoor leadership programs that develop youth communication, confidence, and collaboration.

Outreach that encompasses other topics like drugs and alcohol, academic success, study groups, community service projects, and healthy relationships is needed.

Event evaluation results indicate that youth were impacted in a positive manner and, for most, their expectations were met. Youth were from two rural communities that were part of the same school district. All youth were male, average age 14.3 years (SD = 1.80, range 12–18):

- Seventy percent have a better understanding about youth leadership development.
- Ninety percent would attend more events.

- Seventy-five percent felt the staff were knowledgeable about the topics presented.
- Sixty percent will tell their family and friends about their experience at the event.
- Eighty percent felt the activities were fun and interesting.

The results from the leadership survey and youth quality of life scale indicate that youth feel good about themselves and the friends they have. Most feel that they are getting a good education and can take part in the same activities as other youth. Youth also look forward to the future, and feel that they are important. These statements ranked highest. In comparison, the lowest mean scores are related to feeling alone in life, getting along with parents, and feeling understood by parents.

Recommendations and lessons learned

This section can be combined in an evaluation report or include two stand-alone sections. When you decide how to write the recommendations and lessons learned section, consider your evaluation purpose, your audience, and the primary "takeaway" from the report. When developing recommendations, make sure they align with the evaluation purpose—consider creating a succinct list. Lessons learned accounts of what occurred during the program that might be helpful for future efforts. These are practical statements and may be framed as challenges or solutions (Box 8.5).

BOX 8.5 Field notes on recommendations and lessons learned

Challenges and recommendations

Challenge 1. The focus of youth stress was not appropriate for the intervention and audience.

To begin, the initial proposal sought to understand and document youth stress. The content of the program activities did not focus on stress and healthy coping, but on team work and leadership skills. Recommendation 1. Be flexible in the approach, know the kinds of cultural activities that are planned in advance, and develop measures that assess these activities.

Challenge 2. The initial recruitment goal was not met. The initial recruitment goal was 20 youths aged 13–18 years. A total of 12 youths were

recruited, and participation varied by week. Three youths wanted to participate in the program, but were under the age of 13 and not eligible. Recommendation 2. Over recruit youth or expand the age groups to increase
eligibility.

Challenge 3. Multiple program leaders and directions made it difficult to
focus program efforts.

This program was led by three different people at different times in the
last two years. Each program lead had a different approach and a slightly
different idea about what the youth leadership program should be. Some
of the ideas from previous program leads were incorporated into the current program, but they were difficult to implement. The initial proposal
and timeline was ambitious, given the limited staff time, limited funding,
and the uncertainty about future funding—this program was implemented
in a cautious manner that took into account these factors. Recommendation 3. Even the best ideas can be abandoned if they do not work for the
team.

Conclusion

The results from the youth leadership program underscore the need for more
programming and funding that supports rural youth leadership. Our primary
evaluation questions were answered through the data we collected and analyzed. These may be used by the school, policy makers, funding agency, and
community stakeholders to develop programming.

Dissemination

In the coming months, we will share the results of this initial effort with
our community, the schools, youth participants, and their parents. It is our
hope that these discussions will result in expanding youth leadership programs to reach more youth while promoting resiliency for healthy future
generations.

Now that we have covered the basic components of an evaluation report,
let's review how to communicate and apply evaluation findings for maximum
impact.

Communicating evaluation results

There are four basic elements of a communication model: messages, sources,
channels, and audiences (Nelson et al., 2009). **Messages** are what you use
to communicate the results with the target audience. To communicate messages effectively, use a storyline. Consider these questions, "What is the main

finding (s) of the evaluation?" and "What one message do you want everyone to know?" (Nelson et al., 2009, p. 6). **Sources** may be interpersonal (friends, family members, counselors, or program staff) or mediated (journalists or policy makers).

Channels relate to sources in that the way we share information may involve personal communications or more public approaches. The **audience** we target in communicating evaluation results will vary. Audiences may be from the community, program staff, policy makers, government agencies, fellow evaluators, students, scientists, authors, or reporters and writers.

Recommendations for applying evaluation findings

The primary reason for conducting a program evaluation is to ensure that a dissemination feedback loop exists, so that evaluation results are shared with stakeholders, who use the information to improve their programs and guide future planning efforts (Muller, Burke, Luke, and Harris, 2008, p. 170).

Understanding how to disseminate evaluation results to various program stakeholders, funding agencies, community members, and policy makers is imperative. Previous research on evaluating the effectiveness of evaluation dissemination strategies has found that using multiple dissemination channels to disseminate results helps ensure that they reach their intended audience (Muller et al., 2008). In a study of state tobacco control program evaluation in eight states, each state was assigned a dissemination condition. The first group received print reports only, the second group received reports and the website, the third group received reports and a workshop, and the fourth group received all three dissemination modes. Authors found that participants who used all three dissemination modes were more likely to share results with their colleagues and they found the results more useful than the other groups who did not utilize all three dissemination modes (Muller et al., 2008). Recommendations from this study on disseminating evaluation results have been corroborated by other researchers.

Successful dissemination strategies have three things in common. First, the dissemination approach is tailored to the audience with a focus on the content, key findings or main message, and the medium (written, oral, web-based, others). Second, the source of the message is clear and focused. Third, dissemination promotes an active discussion of the evaluation findings (Keen & Todres, 2007). Active discussions occur with the people, in the place, and with the point of finding meaning and value in the results.

Consider the active dissemination plan (Table 8.1) when answering the following questions:

How results will be disseminated? How will results be used? How will findings affect current and future programs? When results will be available? How do results respond to the community's need/evaluation purpose?

TABLE 8.1 Active Dissemination Plan

Audience	Multiple Dissemination Mediums	Frequency or Date	Responsible Person	Active Follow-up Questions
Health program staff, policy makers, community stakeholders, funding agency	Oral presentations at site coordinator meetings, summary report posted on website, local radio station broadcast, update Facebook page	Beginning of program, quarterly, when updates are available, at the end with key findings and recommendations	Evaluator, program staff, website manager, Facebook page host. Others as appropriate.	How are results used? Who is talking about them? Where do they matter? What is the meaning?

Best practices for disseminating results

Each dissemination approach has strengths and weaknesses that must be considered. There are numerous dissemination mediums that can be used to share evaluation results. These include social media, blog posts, electronic newsletters, website posts and brief updates, radio broadcast, a press release, presentations, reports, and peer-reviewed journal articles (Palen, 2014). Not all rural areas have access to the Internet; this means that dissemination efforts that rely on electronic or web-based mediums may not reach rural populations. Rural areas often have a local radio station, and this can be one way that evaluation results and findings can be shared with the community. Rural areas often have one or two locations that are frequented by the community—gas stations, grocery stores, and churches. These are great places to disseminate evaluation results in various ways—presentation, printed brochure, poster, or printed community paper (local news, local shopper, and others) (Table 8.2).

Every rural community is different, and every data set and source that we use is different—let's take a look at three different approaches used in real-world rural evaluation contexts to answer an evaluation question and report results back to the community.

Computers may not be available in rural settings. Evaluators can work with program staff and stakeholders to access data, enter data into an electronic database or format, analyze results, and report information back to the community. Let's look at a rural evaluation example (Figure 8.2).

Visual images are powerful ways to report the process or impact of a program. We evaluated a school-based recycling program in rural Montana community. We worked with students to document recycling availability and knowledge before the program was implemented, and after the program was in place for six months (Figure 8.3).

TABLE 8.2 Considering the Best Dissemination Approach for Rural Communities

Dissemination Approach	Strengths	Weaknesses	In a Rural Community?
Written report	Easy to access Easy to create	May not reach intended audience Printing costs	Yes
Oral presentation	Increases awareness and support Provides immediate feedback and discussion	May not reach intended audience May not have a venue for the oral presentation	Yes
Press release	Focused message Reaches a lot of people	May not be appropriate Findings may not be newsworthy	Yes
Electronic newsletter	Reaches people with access to Internet No printing costs	May not reach target audience Requires email addresses or access to a website for posting	Sometimes
Social media	YouTube, Facebook, Instagram, Twitter are free and fast. May appeal to younger audiences	May not reach target audience May not be viewed as credible	Sometimes
Journal article	Builds scientific evidence and support for evaluation and recommendations	Target audience may not have access to journal Fees associated with publications may outweigh benefits	Sometimes
Radio/TV broadcast	Reaches unique population. Seeing and hearing individual speak can make message more meaningful May appeal to older audiences	May not be available in some communities. May not reach target audience May be cost prohibitive	Yes

Question: What was the prevalence of diabetes by age and gender during Fiscal Year 2014?

Action Step #1: Local site coordinator worked with clinic to retrieve diabetes data.

Action Step #2: Clinic retrieved data from charts, recorded information on a piece of paper.

Action Step #3: Site coordinator scanned copy of paper to evaluator to enter into MS Excel.

Action Step #4: Evaluator shared MS Excel file with site coordinator and clinic to ensure accuracy.

Action Step #5: Evaluator confirmed accuracy and analyzed data using data provided and 2014 patient population.

Action Step #5: Evaluator reported information back to site coordinator and clinic in a simple, easy to use format with a clear message.

Follow-up: Who received the report? What questions did they have? How well did the report assess prevalence?

FIGURE 8.2 Field Notes on Rural Evaluation Reporting with Limited Computer Access.

Question: Is a school - based recycling program feasible in this rural community?

Action Step #1: Local environmental office worked with schools to determine recycling needs.

Action Step #2: Evaluator interviewed students and teachers to document knowledge, attitudes, and beliefs about recycling efforts. Due to the rural location and costs, the school does not recycle anything. "By the end of the week, our garbage cans are full, recycling would help divert some of the waste and result in a cost-savings for waste transport."- School Administrator

Action Step #3: Environmental office, school, and solid waste department explored feasibility of recycling program using photos, interviews, and administrative reports.

Six-months Later: School applied and received a grant from the USDA to pilot a school-based recycling program. "We used the feasibility report to apply for funding that would support a pilot school-based recycling program."- Stakeholder

Follow-up: What were the strengths and weaknesses of the feasibility report? Was it used during the pilot program?

FIGURE 8.3 Field Notes on Rural School–Based Recycling Program.

Interviews are powerful ways to report perspectives. We implemented a youth drug and alcohol prevention program in a rural South Dakota community. To document youth hopes for the program, we developed an interview guide with a series of questions. Our goal was to solicit feedback from youth about the program and use their feedback to tailor the prevention program approach to meet these needs (Figure 8.4).

Documenting community perspectives, priorities, or feedback in rural settings can be challenging. We partnered with the local school to set up a booth during a basketball game. More than 500 people attended. We used bright colored sticky notes and large pieces of white paper to display attendee responses about the kinds of activities that are needed in the community for youth (Figure 8.5).

Question: What do you hope comes from this prevention program?

Action Step #1: Interview guide developed with input from community, youth, and stakeholders with a focus on the evaluation purpose.

Action Step #2: Evaluator interviewed seven youth to document their hopes for the program and the community.

Action Step #3: Videos were watched, transcribed, and analyzed by the evaluator.

Action Step #4: Initial themes shared with stakeholder group and youth to validate. Report of "hopes" shared to inform program implementation.

Six-months Later: The same seven youth were interviewed again and asked, "What happened as a result of this program?" Steps #3-4 repeated. Data were compared to document how well program achieved student hopes for the program. Results reported.

Follow-up: Who read the initial and follow-up report? In what form? What other themes emerged during the second interview?

FIGURE 8.4 Field Notes on Interviews to Document Impact.

Question: What kinds of youth activities are needed in the community?

Action Step #1: Youth program partnered with local school to set-up a booth at a basketball game.

Action Step #2: Evaluator supported effort, purchased sticky notes and large white poster paper, and markers for written responses.

Action Step #3: To increase participation, everyone who wrote a something on a note received a raffle ticket for a gift card.

Action Step #4: Evaluator and program staff reviewed responses, transcribed into MS Word, uploaded into a qualitative software program, analyzed responses by content analysis and frequency.

Action Step #5: Initial report developed with most frequent responses for youth activities. Brief report shared with program,school, community partners, and youth serving organizations.

Follow-up: What was done with the information? Were data used to establish or improve youth activities?

FIGURE 8.5 Field Notes on Documenting Community Perspectives.

Summary

In this chapter, we have reviewed the basic elements of an evaluation report and dissemination strategies for rural communities. One the most important aspects of developing an evaluation report is developing an evaluation plan first. Understanding context, your target audience, and how the information will be used are critical considerations for evaluation reports. We reviewed several examples of how evaluation data are collected and reported from real-world evaluation practice. These approaches demonstrate the process and flexibility that is needed in rural evaluation contexts. Reporting and dissemination are critical. What good is a report if it is not used, read, and discussed among those who can use the information to improve programs, policies, and effectiveness?

Points to remember

1. Reporting evaluation results is a process that includes the following steps: engage stakeholders, define the audience, plan for dissemination, know the purpose, and report.
2. Evaluation reports, presentations, and communications will include data, often qualitative and quantitative. Know your audience, seek feedback, and make sure your message is reaching those who need to know it.
3. Presenting data effectively requires effort and skills. Know how to communicate your findings for impact.
4. Active dissemination plans require multiple dissemination mediums, frequent communications, and follow-up. Know this and do this.
5. Each dissemination approach has strengths and weaknesses. Know community context and the preferred medium of dissemination based on the message you want to send and your intended audience.

Additional reading and resources

On Evaluation Dissemination Strategies
United Nations Development Fund for Women (2009). *Evaluation Guidance Note Series No.10.* http://www.endvawnow.org/uploads/browser/files/UNIFEM_guidance%20note_evaluation_Dissemination.pdf

On Evaluation Reporting Elements
Centers for Disease Control and Prevention (2013). *Evaluation Reporting: A Guide to Help Ensure Use of Evaluation Findings.* Atlanta, GA: US Department of Health and Human

On Presenting Data
National Cancer Institute (2009) *Making Data Talk: A Workbook. US Department of Health and Human Services National Institutes of Health.* Retrieved from https://www.cancer.gov/publications/health-communication/making-data-talk.pdf

Chapter questions

1. List the components of a basic evaluation report.
2. What are the four main elements of a communication model?
3. Summarize the recommendations for presenting evaluation data effectively in a report.
4. Describe three ways to reach rural audiences with evaluation results?
5. What is the evaluation method that focuses on utilization of findings?
6. Describe the strengths and weaknesses of dissemination approaches in rural communities. Can you think of other mediums that may be used in rural communities? Can you think of mediums that may be used in more rural areas that would not be appropriate for rural communities?

Activities

1. Read the United Nations report on developing an evaluation dissemination strategy (available at: http://www.endvawnow.org/uploads/browser/files/ UNIFEM_guidance%20note_evaluation_Dissemination.pdf). Answer the five evaluation strategy questions as if you are in a rural evaluation context.
2. Create an outline for an evaluation report using the presentation recommendations highlighted in this chapter and the basic components of an evaluation report. What parts of the report are easy to read? What kinds of figures and graphics would you include from your rural evaluation results?

References

Centers for Disease Control and Prevention (2013). *Evaluation reporting: A guide to help ensure use of evaluation findings.* Atlanta, GA: US Department of Health and Human.

Evergreen, S. D. (2017). *Presenting data effectively: Communicating your findings for maximum impact.* Thousand Oaks, CA: Sage Publications.

Keen, S., & Todres, L. (2007). Strategies for disseminating qualitative research findings: Three exemplars. *Forum Qualitative Sozialforschung/Forum: Qualitative Social Research, 8*(3), Art. 17, http://nbn-resolving.de/urn:nbn:de:0114-fqs0703174.

Mueller, N. B., Burke, R. C., Luke, D. A., & Harris, J. K. (2008). Getting the word out: Multiple methods for disseminating evaluation findings. *Journal of Public Health Management and Practice, 14*(2), 170–176.

Nelson, D. E., Hesse, B. W., & Croyle, R. T. (2009). *Making data talk: Communicating public health data to the public, policy makers, and the press.* New York, NY: Oxford University Press.

Palen, L. (2014, July). *Disseminating evaluation results.* Washington, DC: Administration on Children Youth and Families, Family and Youth Services Bureau.

9
PRACTICAL ISSUES FOR RURAL EVALUATORS

There are people that write about evaluation, but do not do evaluation. There are people that do evaluation, but do not write about it. I happen to do both. My goal in writing this chapter is to cover some practical issues that you may experience as a rural evaluator.

Challenges for rural evaluators from the field

Statement of work

We know a statement of work (**SOW**) includes the purpose of the evaluation, the questions that the evaluation will answer, the quality of results, the skills needed, and the time and budget required to support the evaluation (Blue, 2010). **#1 Challenge**—The SOW does not take into account the geographic, social, cultural, political, and technical nuances of our program or population under assessment. **#1 Solution**—SOWs are developed by a program or funding agency. I encourage evaluation practitioners to respond to the SOW and outline areas that need to be revisited for a well-crafted evaluation. **#1 Real-world example**—The SOW was too ambitious. It was developed before the program was funded and by someone who was not familiar with geographic location of the community and the limited technology available. One of the deliverables in the SOW was to develop a website for the program. Because, most community members did not have access to the Internet, traditional web-based marketing methods and communications would not reach the community and target population. The team revised the SOW to include print posters, oral presentations, and local radio station communications rather than web-based marketing strategies.

Preparation and education

#2 Challenge—Training programs may not prepare evaluators to address unique challenges of rural evaluation. **#2 Solution**—Evaluators can overcome this challenge by spending time in rural communities and developing trusting relationships with the population they work with (Green & Haines, 2015; Klitgaard, 2018). **#2 Real-world example**—An environmental program hired an evaluator to complete an evaluation of a solid waste disposal and recycling program. He was surprised that the community lacked solid waste facilities and did not recycle. He was critical in his appraisal of the environmental program and felt the program had failed to serve the community. His lack of cultural responsiveness was noticed by the environmental program director and staff during a meeting. The evaluator apologized to the program staff members and promised to be more culturally responsive in the future.

Local policies and staffing

 # 3 Challenge—Changes in local leadership and staffing turnover impact the ability of the evaluator to complete evaluations. **#3 Solution**—Accept that change is inevitable. Develop a contingency plan for conducting the evaluation (World Health Organization, 2018). Cross-train program staff and other individuals in the community who are involved in the evaluation. **#3 Real-world example**—The community just received funding for a five-year program to prevent youth suicide. Leadership in the community was unstable and this impacted the community's ability to move forward with implementing the program. It took over a year for the leadership to stabilize. The program staff and evaluator kept the funding agency informed and adjusted their implementation time line and goals.

Balancing program needs with funding agency requirements

#4 Challenge—Balancing program evaluation requirements with rural community interests and needs can be difficult. **#4 Solution**—It can be difficult to balance the evaluation needs with the community interests. To overcome this challenge, make sure the evaluation plan or SOW includes input from the community. **#4 Real-world example**—The community wanted to create a video of youth attending a summer camp, but this was not in the program evaluation and the funding agency did not consider videos an acceptable data source. The evaluation team used their phones to create a high-quality video of the youth and posted the videos to the program website. The evaluator helped collect additional data to meet the needs of the funding agency evaluation requirements.

Limited resources

#5 Challenge—Limited resources and staffing require evaluators to wear multiple hats and provide additional program and partner support. **#5**

Solution—The lack of resources and population often means that evaluators will do many things, not just evaluate. Know what you are comfortable with. Set boundaries early and identify other program areas that you may be willing to support. **#5 Real-world example**—The evaluator was asked to meet with a program team who was not part of her evaluation contract. This program was experiencing challenges with data collection and funding agency requirements and asked for her feedback. She was comfortable meeting with the other program and providing guidance without payment.

Overall challenges from published literature

Slow to change

Leviton's article, "Evaluation use: Advances, challenges, and applications" (2003) describes challenges in evaluation ranging from the need for a better standard of evidence, specific guidance on evaluation techniques, the use of social science principles, and the inclusion of context. Leviton argues that little has changed in the evaluation field since 1977 with Michael Quinn Patton's seminal article, "In search of impact: An analysis of the utilization of federal health evaluation research". Leviton feels that evaluators remain largely challenged by the same issues that plagued evaluation 40 years ago. Leviton calls for evaluators to address challenges by focusing on fitting the evaluation findings to the community (2003).

Program theories fail to explain outcomes

Often programs do not work as they are intended (or following a theory)—evaluators lead efforts to determine why. Evaluators may explore the reasons why a program did not work post hoc (Rogers, Petrosino, Huebner, & Hacsi, 2000). However, limited program data limits an evaluator's ability to determine why programs do not work. Another challenge that evaluators experience relates to attributing outcomes to a program (Rogers et al., 2000). Without counterfactual data to support causal attributions, it can be difficult to isolate outcomes caused by a program.

School-based behavioral health program evaluation

Jaycox, McCaffrey, Ocampo, Shelley, Blake, Peterson, Kub, and colleagues explored implementation and outcome evaluation challenges in three separate school-based behavioral health programs (2006). Authors report six common challenges: (1) difficulties with the research design, (2) recruitment issues, (3) protecting participant's privacy, (4) difficulties with implementing the program, (5) cyclical approach of implementation evaluation, and (6) dissemination (Jaycox et al., 2006).

Rural health department evaluation

Beaulieu and Webb (2002) identified several evaluation challenges in rural health departments. First, rural health departments have limited budgets and provide more direct patient services—this challenges evaluation because there are limited staff to evaluate programs. Second, many rural health program staff do not have training or experience in evaluating programs. They are also less likely to have access to evaluation technical assistance when compared with more urban health programs. Third, retaining program staff in rural health departments is an issue—without staff who are familiar with the community, context, and program—it can be difficult to evaluate a program. Participatory evaluation models that utilize community-based research partners rather than external evaluators are helpful in addressing these challenges (Minkler & Wallerstein, 2003).

Implementation of an arthritis campaign in rural Arkansas

Authors Balamurugan, Rivera, Sutphin, and Campbell (2007) implemented an arthritis campaign in rural Arkansas. Limited financial resources meant that communicating information about the program (and results) using television, radio, and print methods were not possible. Another challenge they identified was the hesitancy of some rural staff members to work with other team members from a neighboring metropolitan area. Overall, authors report that limited program staff and the use of program volunteers hindered program reach, follow-up, and evaluation efforts (Balamurugan et al., 2007).

Process evaluation challenges

Previous research demonstrates that local governments, community organizations, and public agencies can have a greater impact if they engage community members frequently and with attention to diversity (Butterfoss, 2006). Some of the challenges that evaluators may experience in process evaluation relate to measuring community participation and promoting community-engaged evaluation practice. Several authors have explored the challenges of community participation in process evaluation and reported that community engagement is hindered when individuals feel they do not have influence over outcomes, they do not receive credit for the work they have done, or they feel their opinions are not valued (Butterfoss, 2006; Kenney & Soafer, 2000; Lasker, Weiss, & Miller, 2001).

Community engagement and support for evaluation is critical, but often the time it takes to fully engage and participate in evaluation is not realistic. To address these challenges, the Center for Rural Pennsylvania developed an eight-step process for engaging citizens (Bassler, Brasier, Fogle, & Taverno, 2008).

BOX 9.1 Developing a rural citizen engagement plan

Step 1: Define the issue. "What is the problem or issue that needs to be addressed?"

Step 2: Identify why citizens should be engaged and their level of engagement. "Why do citizens need to be involved in the program and evaluation?"

Step 3: Find opportunities to engage rural citizens. "What tools can be used to reach rural citizens?" (i.e. surveys, focus groups, public hearings, community task force)

Step 4: Determine who should be involved. "Who needs to be involved in the program / evaluation to accomplish your goals?"

Step 5: Create a plan for recruiting and retaining citizens. "How will you contact and persuade people to be involved in your program/evaluation?" and "How will you retain and reward citizens for their participation?"

Step 6: Ensure a positive environment. "Are meetings effective, conflicts resolved, and citizen ideas valued?"

Step 7: Create benchmarks to track progress. "When will you know that your task has been accomplished?"

Step 8: Communicate. "How will you ensure on-going, regular communications with citizens?"

Source: Bassler, Brasier, Fogle, and Taverno (2008)

TABLE 9.1 Field Notes on Checklist for Making Sure Evaluators Fit Rural Needs

Is the evaluator willing to put the needs of the community and program first and has no hidden agenda?

Can the evaluator communicate effectively and with different people, groups, or organizations involved?

Is the evaluator culturally responsive while respecting the rural community culture and norms?

Does the evaluator treat all team members and community members with respect as equals?

Is the evaluator able to keep information confidential and be ethical?

Is the evaluator committed to the process and community?

What is known about the evaluator's past performance?

Fit

Identifying evaluators that will fit well with the community and evaluation needs is a must. When looking for an external evaluator, rural communities often consider several questions (Table 9.1).

Relationships are critical for rural evaluators. When considering fit, I encourage evaluators to consider what they know, what they think they know, and what communities want to know. Finding balance can help support rural evaluators as they find the best fit for their skills and interests along with rural community needs.

Hiring an evaluator, contracts and agreements

Communities must first determine the type of evaluator that is needed. Community or in-house planners/evaluators may be established to carry out an evaluation. When this occurs, it is useful if at least one member of the team has research and evaluation experience. In-house community evaluators are typically not hired or paid. Contracts or agreements may be developed based on their scope of work and the needs of the program. Professional consultants also serve as evaluators. Often they work with a team of individuals. An example would be a doctoral trained researcher/evaluator who leads evaluation supported by data mangers, administrative assistants, students, and others. Professional consultants will respond to a request for proposals (RFP) or contracts. RFP in general includes the evaluator's salary, data entry, data management, data analyses, report writing, data collection instrument development, pilot testing, and the salaries of individuals who conduct these tasks (Box 9.2).

In contrast, an external evaluator's evaluation contract proposal is targeted at evaluators who are contractors, not employees or internal program evaluators (Box 9.3).

BOX 9.2 Rural program evaluator RFP

Position description

Program Evaluator

Reports to: Epidemiology Manager Supervises: None Salary Grade: CCS 11 FLSA

Classification: Exempt Position Summary: The Program Evaluator will assess the effectiveness and measure the performance of a wide range of health intervention efforts/programs which will be implemented by tribal health programs/entities throughout the state of CA. Additionally, the Program Evaluator will build and maintain effective collaborations with key stake holders including but not limited to Tribal leaders, health providers, tribal health boards and the funding agency.

Essential Functions:

1. Serve as the performance measurement expert.
2. Work effectively with tribes and technical assistance experts to develop a deep understanding of the multifaceted issues revolving around health

promotion and disease prevention and create sustainable strategies for change.

3. Develop, manage and support projects that demand high level quantitative and financial skills to inform strategies, performance objectives, and program results

4. Conduct and produce professional, thorough, rigorous, and insightful analyses and evaluative outputs.

5. Demonstrate working knowledge of and professional experience using statistical evaluation packages, as well as MS Office products.

6. Troubleshoot data-quality issues.

7. Prepare regulatory documents.

8. Other duties as assigned.

Source: Adapted from the American Evaluation Association (2018)

BOX 9.3 External evaluation contract RFP example

Scope of work goals

The Preservation Alliance of West Virginia (PAWV) invites proposals from qualified researchers and consultants to work closely with staff to develop an outcomes-based evaluation plan, process, and tools for the Preserve WV AmeriCorps program based on the program's theory of change, logic model, and performance measures. The time line goal is to complete this project and have the evaluation plan and survey tools ready to implement at the start of the 2017–2018 program year, Monday, August 28, 2017.

PAWV has existing systems and tools for performance measure data collection, storage, processing, analysis, and reporting, but it is soliciting an external evaluator to improve and standardize these systems and tools, as well as create additional evaluation tools to communicate the impact of the Preserve WV AmeriCorps program with the grantor and general public.

Deadlines

By Friday, March 10, by 5:00 p.m. EST, potential bidders should email the project coordinator with a brief, initial statement of interest in bidding. The project coordinator will then email potential bidders the full RFP containing all relevant information.

Questions from bidders must be submitted by email to project coordinator by Wednesday, March 15, by 5:00 p.m. EST. All relevant questions and responses will be compiled and emailed to all known bidders by Monday, March 20.

Proposals must be emailed to project coordinator, date- and time-stamped by 5:00 p.m. EST on Friday, March 24, 2017.
Award Date: Friday, April 7, 2017

Source: Preserve West Virginia (2017)

Cost of rural evaluation

Evaluators may be involved in developing a budget for a rural program; in other instances, they may be hired after a program is funded and there is a set amount in the budget for the evaluation—costs for evaluation vary considerably. The Corporation for National and Community Service (CNCS) reviewed 16 nonexperimental evaluation budgets and calculated the median evaluation budgets—the median evaluation budget per year for nonexperimental evaluations was $40,700 and, for quasi-experimental design, evaluations were similar at $38,434 (ND). Authors report that 13%–15% of the program budget should be allocated for evaluation with nonexperimental designs and quasi-experimental designs, and the percentage increased to 20%. For randomized control trails, the percentage of the budget generally exceeds 25% (CNCS, ND). When considering costs, keep in mind the type of evaluation that is required, the skill level that is needed, the costs of travel to and from the community, the evidence required, and the number of staff required to carry out an evaluation.

Other cost considerations

There are five considerations when developing a rural program budget. First, transportation costs may be higher for program staff, community members, and the contractual staff (evaluator). Second, if the community has an emerging infrastructure and limited computers, office space, office furniture, and general office supplies, the first-year budget should include these items and, in subsequent years, they should be budgeted as needed. Third, professional printing costs for reports and brochures generated through a program/evaluation may be higher due to shipping costs associated with the rural community. Fourth, travel for contacts (training, services, evaluation, and marketing coordination) may be higher in rural communities. Hotel accommodations may not be available in the same town, this means that travel should include extra mileage to travel to and from hotels. Many rural communities do not have airports, rental car locations, and restaurants—these factors increase travel costs and should be planned for in the budget.

Budget examples and definitions may not apply to every program or organization. Federal, state, local, and private funders of rural programs often have specific budgetary guidance that should be reviewed and adhered to when developing a rural program budget. Most federal grants have specific allowable costs. Federal cost principles are outlined in 2 Code of Federal Regulations (CFR) Parts 225, 220, and 230. Most funding agencies outline funding limitations for data collection and performance assessment. These costs are typically averaged across time for multiyear grants, and in some cases, costs cannot exceed 20% of the total budget period (Substance Abuse and Mental Health Services Administration, 2018).

Opportunities for rural evaluators

Evaluation findings may address other areas and disciplines not directly related to the program.

One emerging area of interest across program disciplines is the social determinants of health (SDOH). The SDOH are conditions of place, where people live, grow old, die, work, and play (Marmot et al., 2008). Evaluation of programs in rural communities may identify factors like economic stability, neighborhood and physical environment, education, food, community and social context, and health care systems. These determinants lead to health outcomes that are an important focus area for many rural programs.

Social change

Rural evaluators are in a unique position to impact social change. Global evaluations with US Agency for International Development (USAID), the World Health Organization, and the European Union demonstrate the power of evaluation to impact social change. Examples of evaluation that have impacted social change include: sustained changes in behaviors about health, supporting health care workers and barriers to care, building capacity of organizations to implement social behavior change interventions (USAID, 2018). Rural-focused evaluation supports the improvement of key determinants that impact health (Figure 9.1).

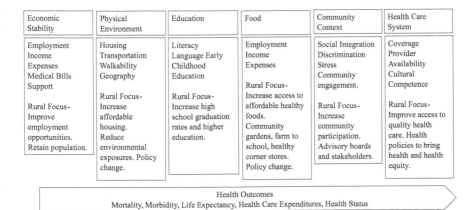

Economic Stability	Physical Environment	Education	Food	Community Context	Health Care System
Employment Income Expenses Medical Bills Support	Housing Transportation Walkability Geography	Literacy Language Early Childhood Education	Employment Income Expenses	Social Integration Discrimination Stress Community engagement.	Coverage Provider Availability Cultural Competence
Rural Focus-Improve employment opportunities. Retain population.	Rural Focus-Increase affordable housing. Reduce environmental exposures. Policy change.	Rural Focus-Increase high school graduation rates and higher education.	Rural Focus-Increase access to affordable healthy foods. Community gardens, farm to school, healthy corner stores. Policy change.	Rural Focus-Increase community participation. Advisory boards and stakeholders.	Rural Focus-Improve access to quality health care. Health policies to bring health and health equity.

Health Outcomes
Mortality, Morbidity, Life Expectancy, Health Care Expenditures, Health Status

FIGURE 9.1 Evaluation and the Social Determinants of Health in Rural Communities. *Source*: Adapted from Artiga and Hinton (2018).

BOX 9.4 Field notes on rural evaluator opportunities

We put in a data request to the local clinic that would allow us to examine prevalence in substance use over a four-year period. We received the data and then analyzed the results. As a team, we reviewed the results and talked about what they meant. We also reviewed the results as a way of checking the validity of data. For example, for one year, the substance use prevalence for adults aged 18 and over was 15%. This seemed high since the substance use prevalence in the United States was 8%. However, after reviewing other data sources and talking with community members and program staff, we agreed that this prevalence was probably accurate.

The Board of Directors gave us permission to share results with other community programs. We developed easy-to-read reports with prevalence data and written recommendations on how our program was going to address these recommendations to decrease substance use prevalence. Since we work in a small rural community, most offices do not have a data manager or anyone generating reports about the prevalence of substance use. This was a unique opportunity to share information about substance use prevalence with other programs in the community.

Workforce development

Another opportunity for rural evaluators is to help train and develop the workforce. This can be in areas of evaluation, data entry, computer skills, oral and written communications, and program planning. Evaluators can reach other programs and people through their efforts (Box 9.4).

Education and professional associations

It is easy to get so wrapped up in evaluation that we do not take time to sharpen our skills and connect with other evaluators.

Claremont Evaluation Center hosts a variety of professional development workshops and continuing education courses (https://research.cgu.edu/claremont-evaluation-center/professional-development-workshops/). Local universities, community colleges, and state/local programs may sponsor continuing education for rural evaluators as well. Annual conferences like the American Evaluation Association, the American Public Health Association, and the Council for State and Territorial Epidemiologists often include pre- or post-evaluation workshops. Federal agencies like the Environmental Protection Agency, the United States Department of Health and Human Services, and others regularly provide webinars, workshops, and education for evaluators.

Evaluators need to be aware of the best ways to communicate evaluation results. We learned in Chapter 8 that if we want people to read reports, we need to use multiple mediums and find ways to actively discuss the results with our stakeholders and intended audience. To build new skills, consider taking a class, learn a new software program, watch a YouTube video, or purchase a book and teach yourself something new.

Join a professional association; the American Evaluation Association (AEA) has more than 7,300 members from all 50 states and 80 foreign countries. AEA is dedicated to the application of program evaluation and other types of evaluation to improve practice and effectiveness. One of the great things that AEA offers is the AEA 365 Tip A day by and for evaluators. This blog has real-world evaluation scenarios, tips, and resources that can help you become the best rural evaluator that you can be. Standard membership fees are just $100 per year and membership allows you access to a variety of different resources, training opportunities, and networks that can support you and your work (http://www.eval.org).

Summary

In this chapter, we have reviewed some common challenges in evaluation and practical issues from rural community evaluation. There are several challenges that rural evaluators may encounter, but these challenges have solutions. Costs associated with rural evaluation must be considered. Finding a good fit for the evaluator and a program is critical. Sharpening our skills as evaluators is something that we must do. In a constantly changing landscape of technology, travel, budget needs, and communication methods, we must strive to be the best that we can be. Networking with professional organizations like the American Evaluation Association is one of the many resources available for rural evaluators.

Points to remember

1. Rural evaluators will experience challenges, but these are not unsurmountable.
2. The context of rural America is unique—evaluators must attend to culture.
3. For every challenge, there is a solution—community members are often the ones with the solutions. Strengthening partnerships with community members, programs, and leaders will help rural evaluators when they encounter difficulties.
4. Unique opportunities abound in rural evaluation—train the workforce, take a class on how to design a website, and teach a non-evaluator about evaluation—these are just some of the ways that rural evaluators can make a difference.
5. Join a professional association like American Evaluation Association and seek opportunities to refine your evaluation skills, meet new people, and plan for the future.

Additional readings and resources

On American Evaluation Association
AEA 365 Tip A day by and for Evaluators, Retrieved from http://aea365.org/blog/

On Rural Evaluation Challenges
Rural Health Information Hub (2018). Toolkits. Retrieved from https://www.ruralhealthinfo.org/toolkits/rural-toolkit/4/evaluation-challenges

On the Evaluation Statement of Work
Blue, R. (2010). *Preparing and Evaluation Statement of Work (SOW), Performance Monitoring & Evaluation TIPS*, Washington DC, USAID. Retrieved from http://pdf.usaid.gov/pdf_docs/pnadw103.pdf

On Developing a Federal Program Budget
National Institutes of Health (2018). *Develop Your Budget.* https://grants.nih.gov/grants/how-to-apply-application-guide/format-and-write/develop-your-budget.htm

Chapter questions

1. List three challenges that rural evaluators experience. How might you take action to overcome these challenges?
2. Describe the unique opportunities of rural evaluation. Can you think of others? How are these opportunities different than non-rural evaluation?
3. Summarize the basic components of a program budget. In what category would an external evaluator fit under? What are some costs that the evaluator may incur? In what instances would the costs be covered by the program budget? In what instances would the evaluator need to cover these costs?
4. Review the two program evaluators' request for applicants in this chapter. What are some of the differences in qualifications and standards for the internal program evaluator at the California Rural Indian Health Board and the external contract evaluator for the Preserve Alliance in West Virginia?

Practice

1. Go to the AEA 365 Blog website (https://aea365.org/blog/). Search the terms, rural evaluation. List the articles that include tips for conducting evaluation in rural communities. Summarize these articles and describe the "Rad Resources" included for each article.
2. Review 2 CFR 225 Cost principles for state, local, and tribal governments (https://www.gpo.gov/fdsys/granule/CFR-2012-title2-vol1/CFR-2012-title2-vol1-part225/content-detail.html). What are the general principles for determining allowable costs? How might evaluation costs be justified using

these cost principles? Can you think of instances when an evaluator's costs would not be justified?
3. Create a rural program evaluation budget. What did you include and why? Are these costs justified?

References

American Evaluation Association (2018). *Rural evaluation jobs*, Retrieved from http://www.eval.org/p/cm/ld/fid=113

Artiga, S., & Hinton, E. (2018) *Beyond Health Care: The role of social determinants in promoting health and health equity. Kellogg Foundation, Disparities Policy.* Retrieved from http://files.kff.org/attachment/issue-brief-beyond-health-care

Balamurugan, A., Rivera, M., Sutphin, K., & Campbell, D. (2007). Health communications in rural America: Lessons learned from an arthritis campaign in rural Arkansas. *The Journal of Rural Health, 23*(3), 270–275. doi:10.1111/j.1748-0361.2007. 00101.x

Bassler, A., Brasier, K., Fogle, N., & Taverno, R. (2008). *Developing effective citizen engagement: A how-to guide for community leaders. Pennsylvania State University Cooperative Extension April 2008.* Retrieved from http://www.rural.palegislature.us/effective_citizen_engagement.pdf

Beaulieu, J., & Webb, J. (2002). Challenges in evaluating rural health programs. *The Journal of Rural Health, 18*(2), 281–285.

Blue, R. (2010) *Preparing and evaluation Statement of Work (SOW), performance monitoring & evaluation TIPS.* Washington DC: USAID. Retrieved from http://pdf.usaid.gov/pdf_docs/pnadw103.pdf

Butterfoss, F. (2006). Process evaluation for community participation. *Annual Review of Public Health, 27*, 323–340. doi:10.1146/annurev.publhealth.27.021405.102207

Corporation for National and Community Service (ND). *Effectively budgeting for an evaluation overview.* Retrieved from https://www.nationalservice.gov/sites/default/files/resource/Budgeting%20for%20Evaluation%20Description%20of%20video.pdf

Green, G. P., & Haines, A. (2015). *Asset building & community development.* Thousand Oaks, CA: Sage Publications.

Jaycox, L. H., McCaffrey, D. F., Ocampo, B. W., Shelley, G. A., Blake, S. M., Peterson, D. J. ... Kub, J. E. (2006). Challenges in the evaluation and implementation of school-based prevention and intervention programs on sensitive topics. *American Journal of Evaluation, 27*(3), 320–336.

Kenney, E., & Sofaer, S. (2000). *The Coalition Self-Assessment Survey: A manual for users.* New York, NY: School of Public Affairs, Baruch College.

Klitgaard, R. (2018). Evaluation of, for, and through partnerships. In Osvaldo N. Feinstein (Ed.), Chapter 5. *Evaluation and development* (pp. 43–58). New York, NY: Routledge.

Lasker, R. D., Weiss, E. S., & Miller, R. (2001). Partnership synergy: a practical framework for studying and strengthening the collaborative advantage. *The Milbank Quarterly, 79*(2), 179–205. doi:10.1111/1468-0009.00203

Leviton, L. C. (2003). Evaluation use: Advances, challenges and applications. *American Journal of Evaluation, 24*(4), 525–535.

Marmot, M., Friel, S., Bell, R., Houweling, T., Taylor, S., & Commission on Social Determinants of Health (2008). Closing the gap in a generation: health equity through action on the social determinants of health. *The Lancet, 372*(9560), 1661–1669.

Minkler, M., & Wallerstein, N. (2003). *Part one: Introduction to community-based participatory research. Community-based participatory research for health* (pp. 5–24). San Francisco, CA: Jossey-Bass.

Patton, M. (1977). In search of impact: An analysis of the utilization of federal health evaluation research. In C. H. Weiss (Ed.), *Using social re-search in public policy making.* Lexington, MA: Lexington Books.

Preserve West Virginia (2017). *Request for external evaluation contract proposals*, Retrieved from https://preservationalllliancewv.wordpress.com/2017/02/23/request-for-external-evaluation-contract-proposals/

Rogers, P. J., Petrosino, A., Huebner, T. A., & Hacsi, T. A. (2000). Program theory evaluation: Practice, promise, and problems. *New Directions for Evaluation, 2000*(87), 5–13.

Substance Abuse and Mental Health Services Administration (2018). *State-wide family network funding opportunity announcement.* No. SM-18-007, CFDA: 93.243. Retrieved from https://www.samhsa.gov/grants/grant-announcements/sm-18-007

USAID (2018). *Global health: Social and behavior change.* Retrieved from https://www.usaid.gov/what-we-do/global-health/cross-cutting-areas/social-and-behavior-change

World Health Organization (2018). *WHO guidance for contingency planning* (No. WHO/WHE/CPI/2018.13). World Health Organization. Geneva, Switzerland. Retrieved from http://apps.who.int/iris/handle/10665/260554

10

SUSTAINABILITY AND FINAL THOUGHTS FOR RURAL EVALUATORS

What I have come to know about sustainability is that nearly all programs have something that is sustained, even after the funding or program ends. At times sustainability is about changes in behavior, attitudes, ideas, or practices. In other instances, it is about funding to continue a program or continued collaboration. Evaluators help facilitate an important process of determining what should be sustained once a program ends. After the priorities are set, it is just a matter of taking action to ensure that sustainability occurs.

Sustaining outcomes

Defining sustainability

Sustainability is a method of using a resource, so that it is not depleted or permanently changed (Merriam Webster, 2018). Programs, communities, and funding agencies have varied definitions of sustainability.

The Centers for Disease Control defines sustainability as "A community's on-going capacity and resolve to work together to establish, advance, and maintain effective strategies that continuously improve health and quality of life for all" (2013, p. 8).

The Substance Abuse and Mental Health Services Administration (SAMHSA) defines prevention program sustainability as, "…developing prevention systems that promote and support the delivery of effective prevention strategies in order to prevent and reduce substance use, misuse and abuse among whole populations. Ultimately, sustainability is about maintaining positive outcomes in these populations" (2012, para. 1).

The Department of Housing Urban Development calls for an expanded definition of program sustainability:

> Program sustainability has traditionally been viewed as the act of decreasing dependence on one source of funding and shifting financial support for program implementation to a new funding stream. In reality, program and organizational sustainability is a much more complex and dynamic process
>
> *(ND, p. 159)*

Most people think of sustainability as continued funding to support rural programming; however, sustainability also relates to momentum, pooling community resources, and ensuring policies and practices are in place. The Centers for Disease Control writes, "Sustainability is not just about funding. It's about creating and building momentum to maintain communitywide change by organizing and maximizing community assets and resources. It means institutionalizing policies and practices within communities and organizations" (2011, p. 7). As rural evaluators it is essential to create a shared understanding and definition of sustainability with community (Table 10.1).

TABLE 10.1 Program Sustainability Framework Domains and Definitions

Domain	Definition	Rural Considerations
Political/environmental support	Having internal and external support	Gain support early, establish a community advisory board and engage leaders
Funding stability	Establishing a consistent financial base	Multiple funding streams may be necessary, pool resources, and plan funding early
Partnerships	Developing relationships with community, program, and stakeholders	Identify programs with similar goals and mission, invite them to the table and ensure non-duplication of program effort
Organizational capacity	Having support and resources needed to effectively implement and manage	Build organizational capacity early, cross train staff, and develop skills
Program evaluation	Assessing the program to inform planning and document results	Tailor evaluation to the rural context and culture
Program adaptation	Taking actions to adapt or modify program to ensure it continues	Be flexible and willing to fit within the rural context
Communications	Communicating with community and stakeholders in a strategic way	Know how people access information, preferred communication challenges, and what is culturally/linguistically appropriate
Strategic planning	Using a processes to guide a program's directions, goals, and strategies	Begin early, engage community so that they are supportive of the plan and see the benefit

Source: Adapted from Calhoun et al. (2014).

What is a sustainability plan?

A sustainability action plan outlines the steps that are needed to implement a sustainability plan. These priority areas include definitions from Table 10.1. There are numerous approaches to developing a sustainability action plan, and this is just one (Table 10.2).

The Community Tool Box provides a practical guide for sustainability planning in community initiatives and organizations (2018). This guide provides a five-step process for developing a sustainability plan. First determine if the program needs to be sustained and for how long. Next clarify the goals of the program and what actions are needed. Then create a plan that outlines the resources that are needed. Identify what tactics will be used to sustain the program and plan to secure additional resources. Finally, outline a specific action plan for each of the program goals and activities as a result of the sustainability planning effort.

The Centers for Disease Control (CDC) offers a more in-depth process for sustainability planning of health programs. The CDC planning process includes ten steps (Table 10.3).

The Program Sustainability Assessment Tool (PSAT) outlines a three-step process for sustainability planning (Luke, Calhoun, Robichaux, Elliott, & Moreland-Russel, 2014). Luke and colleagues developed the PSAT and tested it with 252 state and community public health programs—this effort resulted in a new instrument that measures sustainability across eight domains (2015). Based on the PSAT, the first step in developing a sustainability action plan is to prepare and assess the program. Second, develop a suitability action plan, and third, take action. In the first step, authors recommend defining the program, initiative, or policy to be sustained and completing the PSAT (https://sustaintool.org/understand/). The second step involves a planning team, knowing the mission and purpose, reviewing assessment results, and determining which program elements or activities need to be sustained. In the third step, communities take action and implement the action plan then reassess sustainability each year. PSAT has been used in various community settings (Luke et al., 2014).

TABLE 10.2 Field Notes on Sustainability Action Plan

Priority Area (Select Three or Less)	Action Steps	Person Responsible	Resources and Stakeholders Required	Methods to Track Progress/Due Date
Partnerships Funding communications Organizational capacity Program adaptation Strategic planning Environmental support Evaluation	What will be done?	Who will do this?	What support is needed?	How will you know it is done? What is the due date?

TABLE 10.3 Ten-step Sustainability Plan for Community Coalitions

Sustainability Steps 1–10	*Rural Considerations*
1. Create a shared definition of sustainability	Shared definitions should include perspectives from multiple programs, partners, and community stakeholders
2. Create a plan	Identify who will coordinate, facilitate, and plan. Create a realistic timeline for completing the sustainability plan
3. Position efforts to increase likelihood of sustainability	Consider current goals, future needs, practices, and funds needed
4. Examine current and pending efforts	Review current program efforts and pending efforts
5. Develop criteria to determine which efforts will continue	Consider importance, feasibility, and evaluation
6. Prioritize efforts	Prioritize efforts based on diverse perspectives. Explore potential successes, barriers, partnerships, evidence, and impact. Leverage existing resources when possible.
7. Maintain priority efforts	Review funding available. Consider when program funding begins and ends. Leverage funds and garner support to maintain priority efforts.
8. Develop a plan to sustain priority efforts (a sustainability plan)	Select one or two members to write the plan based on steps 1–7.
9. Implement sustainability plan	Identify who will lead each priority effort, determine due dates, resources needed, communication required, and steps taken.
10. Evaluate outcomes and revise	Identify areas for improvement and revise plan as necessary.

Source: Adapted from Centers for Disease Control Sustainability Planning Guide (2011).

Another resource for developing sustainability plans is through the routinization or institutionalization of programs. The concept of **routinization**, a process that establishes social activities on a durable basis (Pluye, Potvin, & Dennis, 2004, p. 123), was first introduced in the 1920s by Max Weber. Routinization was further explored by Yin in 1979 using organizational systems that address five areas: budget, personnel, supply and maintenance, training, and organizational governance (Yin, 1979; Yin, 1981). Yin's work on routinization focused on passages where an organization's degree of routinization is assessed using a scale of marginal, moderate, or high points (1979). Since 1979, there have been several sustainability models introduced (Calhoun, et al., 2014; CDC, 2011; Goodman, McLeroy, Steckler, & Hoyle, 1993); however, Yin's Routinization Framework continues to be a widely used tool to assess sustainability (1979).

What factors influence sustainability?

Mary Ann Scheirer (2005) conducted a review of empirical studies to explore program sustainability. Of the 19 studies identified in American and Canadian health programs, 14 continued program activities after the programming ended (Scheirer, 2005). Five factors influenced sustainability: (1) modifying program over time, (2) a local champion (leader), (3) program fit with organization and mission, (4) perceived benefits of a program, and (5) the support of stakeholders and other programs (Scheirer, 2005) (Figure 10.1).

The Healthy Schools/Healthy Students initiative is one example of a national evaluation that explored factors that predict sustainability. This mixed-methods evaluation found that partnerships, sharing resources and funds, advisory committees, and ease of implementation were most predictive of sustainability (Box 10.1).

The Health Resources Services Administration (HRSA) conducted a qualitative evaluation of 102 previous grantees in rural and urban areas. HRSA found that the dynamics of sustainability involve leadership, relevance and value of program, reasons for working together, and how sustainability programs are established (2012). HRSA recommends using three questions to review program sustainability (2012, p. 9).

1. What has been sustained?
2. What has not been sustained?
3. What led to these results?

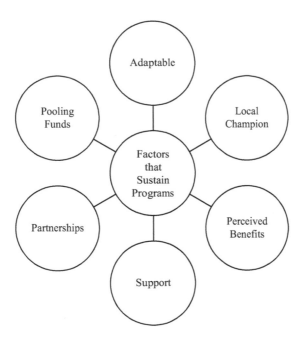

FIGURE 10.1   Factors That Sustain Rural Programs.
Source: Based on Schrier (2005) and SAMHSA (2012).

BOX 10.1 The healthy schools initiative, factors that predict sustainability

Background: The National Evaluation of the Safe Schools/Healthy Students (SS/HS) Initiative explored factors that predict grantee sustainability in more than 365 school districts in the United States.

   Evaluation Question: What factors predict sustainability in SS/HS grantees?

   Methods: The national cross-site evaluation utilized a combination of methodological approaches to explore patterns in sustainability across grantees and data sources. Data included web-based survey data from grantees, site visits data, annual outcome data, phone interviews, Census data, in-person interviews, and Government Performance Results Act (GPRA) data.

   Analyses: Descriptive statistics, meta-analysis of GPRA data using meta-regression focusing on 12-GPRA outcome measures, and multilevel growth curve modeling.

   Results: Authors report that by the end of the third year, 93 percent of the grantees had established strong collaboration among local stakeholders, and 95 percent had established a reputation for effectiveness. Multiple factors were associated with sustainability, these include: well-established partnerships at the beginning of the program, pooling funds among several programs and grants, development of advisory committees, and grantees who reported few barriers.

Source: SAMHSA (2013)

These questions may be asked six months after a program ends, or in extreme cases 30 or more years. With a basic understanding of sustainability and factors that influence sustainability, let's examine sustained impacts of rural programs.

Sustained impacts

Sustained impacts are "long-term effects that may or may not be dependence on the continuation of a program" (HRSA, 2012, p. 8). Sustained impacts are not always considered because they are not obvious, and they may not directly tie back to a program or service. Examples of sustained impacts include improvements in collaboration, service, capacity, policy, knowledge, and behaviors (Figure 10.1).

Evaluation methods that focus on sustainability and impacts

Sustained Emerging Impacts Evaluation (SEIE) is an evaluation method that "examines the extent to which intended impacts have been sustained as well as what unintended impacts have emerged over time, both positive and negative" (Cekan, Zivetz, & Rogers, 2016, para. 2). This method is also called post-project impact evaluation. Typically, SEIEs are conducted 2–10 years after a program has ended, although in some cases 30 years. The process for SEIE is similar to evaluation planning discussed earlier in this book. Let's briefly explore the process. First, develop program theory of change, and this includes a theory of sustainability. Second, determine what success looks like using participatory approach. Next, describe impacts and understand causes. Finally, share results and report information back to agencies, stakeholders, local partners, communities, and governments (Cekan et al., 2016). Plan-international.org reports an example of a sustained impact, "Plan had played a major role in providing physical inputs which are still intact and in use, such as water tanks and new improved latrines" (2012, p. 2). The sustained impact evaluation completed nine years after the program ended found that many of the investments were sustained.

Funding future work

Funding is just one aspect of sustainability, and it happens to be the one that we think about the most. Table 10.4 summarizes funding strategies, potential funding sources, and action steps required to meet the funding need based on a rural community alcohol and drug prevention program.

TABLE 10.4 Field Notes on Funding Strategies, Sources, and Actions

Strategies	Potential Funding Sources	Actions Steps
Local fundraisers 10%=$30,000	Bake sale, garage sale, or car wash	Partner with local community members, businesses, and schools
City or county budget 15% = $45,000	County commissioners, local leaders, or county programs	Develop relationships with county commissioners, attend meetings, and provide updates on prevention needs and activities
In-kind contributions 25%=$75,000	Time donated by programs and volunteers, facilities donated for prevention events, food and supplies donated by businesses	Track in-kind contributions and acknowledge individuals and businesses.
Grants 50% = $150,000	Federal grants Substance Abuse and Mental Health Services Administration (SAMHSA), state and university grants (small), local county grants, local foundation grants	Identify grants that fund prevention activities, and write and submit applications
Goal: $300,000.00		

Utilizing evaluation for policy change and community transformation

Evaluation findings are powerful, and they give a voice to the people and context while influencing policy, social planning, social justice, and transformation. A **policy** is a law, regulation, procedure, action, incentive, or voluntary practice of communities, governments, or other institutions (CDC, 2014). **Policy evaluations** utilize systematic data collection and analysis methods to make decisions about the policy process. Policy enactment, adoption, implementation, update, and enforcement are often short-term outcomes highlighted in the program logic model (if the focus is on policy). Program evaluations may target specific policies, or identify short- and long-term outcomes and impacts related to policy uptake.

Social planning is a process that helps communities identify their resources and needs to improve their quality of life. Evaluators may support social planning through systems, policy, community development, policy analysis, building consensus, awareness and education, and advocacy and action (Community Tool Box, 2018). Today, nearly every rural evaluation requires some aspect of community participation. Community participation has led to transformation and policy change. Examples of policy change based on evaluation findings include primary seat belt enforcement laws (Dinh-Zarr et al., 2001), the Liveable Streets policy in Unionville Missouri (Windmoller, 2013), rural and small-town smart growth initiatives and policies (United States Environmental Protection Agency, 2014), and special education policy changes for English Language Learners (Barrio, 2017). These examples leveraged evaluation findings to support programs and improved policies in rural America. Most policy is informed by evaluation or a needs assessment that documents what is happening and what needs to be changed.

Summary

In this chapter, we have reviewed sustainability and discussed some final thoughts about program evaluation in rural communities. We know that evaluation can be a powerful tool to promote social change and that policies are influenced, created, and sustained through effective program evaluation efforts. Community transformation is possible through rural program evaluation, and the case examples, field notes, publications, and reports highlighted throughout this text are the evidence. You are the vehicle that makes rural evaluation possible.

Final thoughts

There are five reasons why a rural-focused evaluation is needed (Box 10.2).

Evaluation is a tool that can promote social change in rural contexts. We know the importance of a rural-focused evaluation across disciplines, communities, and

---

BOX 10.2 Five reasons to evaluate in rural communities

1—Evaluations tell us what works and what does not work—a must for rural communities.
2—Evaluations can demonstrate the effectiveness of a rural program.
3—Evaluations can improve rural programming and practice across disciplines.
4—Evaluations increase capacity for future work in rural communities.
5—Evaluations build knowledge for current and future generations.

Source: Adapted from USDPHHS (2016)

---

cultures in the United States. This book is an invitation to you—walk through the doors of rural evaluation and see what kind of difference you can make.

The door is wide open, don't go back to sleep

Rumi

Points to remember

1. The time to begin thinking about sustainability is when a program begins (rather than when it ends).
2. Sustainability is not just about funding, sustainability is about determining priorities and finding ways to sustain these priorities over time.
3. There are five factors that influence sustainability—know these and use these.
4. Evaluators should use evaluation to support social planning and policy change.
5. Rural evaluators support informed decision-making, policy change, documenting effectiveness, communicating information, and growing community leaders and champions.

Additional readings and resources

On Sustainability Toolkits
Substance Abuse Mental Health Services Administration Health Research Services Administration *Health Clinic Sustainability* (ND). Retrieved from https://www.integration.samhsa.gov/financing/sustainability

Substance Abuse Mental Health Services Administration (ND). *Planning and Sustainability.* Retrieved from http://captus.samhsa.gov/access-resources/planning-sustainability

Health Resources and Services Administration (2012). *Dynamics of Sustainability.* Department of Health and Human Resources. Retrieved from https://www.ruralhealthinfo.org/assets/1211-4984/dynamics-of-sustainability.pdf

Housing and Urban Development (ND). *Sustainability*. Retrieved from https://www.hud.gov/sites/documents/HHPGM_FINAL_CH7.PDF

USAID Project Starter Resources (ND). *Resources* Retrieved from http://usaidprojectstarter.org/sites/default/files/resources/pdfs/SEC-revised.pdf

On Program Sustainability
Center for Public Health Systems Science (2018). *Washington University in St. Louis. Program Sustainability Assessment Tool*. Retrieved from https://sustaintool.org/understand/

Schroeder, D. (2007). *Sustainability Evaluation: A Checklist Approach Interdisciplinary Evaluation Western Michigan University Evaluation Café*, October 23, 2007 presentation. Retrieved from http://www.wmich.edu/sites/default/files/attachments/u58/2014/cafe-schroeter_slides-Fall-2007.pdf

Program Sustainability Assessment Tool (ND). Retrieved from https://sustaintool.org/understand/

On Sustained Impact Evaluation
Cekan, J., Zivetz, L., and Rogers, P. (2016). *Sustained and Emerging Impacts Evaluation. BetterEvaluation*. Retrieved from http://betterevaluation.org/themes/SEIE

On Funding for Sustaining Programs
Regional Prevention Partnership Sustainability Training (2016). *Sustainability Training Workbook Version 1.1*. Retrieved from http://healthandlearning.org/wp-content/uploads/2015/04/2016-12-7-VT-Sustainability-Training-Workbook-v.1.pdf

On Guiding Program Evaluation
Administration for Children and Families (2016). The Program Managers Guide to Evaluation (2016). Retrieved from https://www.acf.hhs.gov/sites/default/files/opre/program_managers_guide_to_eval2010.pdf

On Policy Change and Evaluation
Centers for Disease Control (2014). *Using Evaluation to Inform CDC's Policy Process*. Atlanta, GA: Centers for Disease Control and Prevention, US Department of Health and Human Services. Retrieved from https://www.cdc.gov/policy/analysis/process/docs/usingevaluationtoinformcdcspolicyprocess.pdf

On Social Planning
Community Tool Box (2018). *Section 3. Social Planning and Policy Change. Chapter 5*. Retrieved from https://ctb.ku.edu/en/table-of-contents/assessment/promotion-strategies/social-planning-policy-change/main

Chapter questions

1. In your own terms, define sustainability. What does it mean, how do rural evaluators plan for sustainability? Why is it important?
2. Summarize CDC's ten-step guide for developing a sustainability plan. Tailor this plan to fit a rural program's need.

3. Describe the three basic steps to Program Sustainability used in the Program Sustainability Assessment Tool.

Practice

1. Go to the Community Tool Box website (https://ctb.ku.edu/en/sustaining-work-or-initiative). Review the section on sustainability. Review the examples by clicking on the tab to the right of the outline. Summarize what these examples have in common. Identify the goals and contexts and how these relate to sustainability planning.
2. Review the Program Managers Guide to Evaluation. List three sections that you would add to this guide based on the information presented in this book. Consider context, culture, and capacity.
3. Go to the Program Sustainability Assessment Tool website (https://sustaintool.org/understand/). Review resources provided on environmental support resources, funding stability, partnerships, organizational capacity, communications, strategic planning, and program evaluation. Select one of the resources and summarize how these might be used in a rural evaluation context.

References

Barrio, B. (2017). Addressing the disproportionality of English language learners in special education programs in rural communities. *Rural Special Education Quarterly, 36*(2), 64–72. doi:10.1177/8756870517707217

Cekan, J., Zivetz, L., & Rogers, P. (2016). *Sustained and emerging impacts evaluation. Better Evaluation.* Retrieved from http://betterevaluation.org/themes/SEIE

Centers for Disease Control (2014). *Using evaluation to inform CDC's policy process.* Atlanta, GA: Centers for Disease Control and Prevention, US Department of Health and Human Services. Retrieved from https://www.cdc.gov/policy/analysis/process/docs/usingevaluationtoinformcdcspolicyprocess.pdf

Centers for Disease Control and Prevention (2011). *CDC's healthy communities program: A sustainability planning guide for healthy communities,* Atlanta, GA: Centers for Disease Control and Prevention, US Department of Health and Human Services, p. 1. Retrieved from http://www.cdc.gov/healthycommunitiesprogram/pdf/sustainability_guide.pdf

Community Tool Box (2018). *Section 3. Social planning and policy change. Chapter 5.* Retrieved from https://ctb.ku.edu/en/table-of-contents/assessment/promotion-strategies/social-planning-policy-change/main

Community Tool Box (2018). *Sustaining the Work or Initiative.* Retrieved from https://ctb.ku.edu/en/sustaining-work-or-initiative

Department of Housing and Urban Development (ND). *Program sustainability.* Retrieved from https://www.hud.gov/sites/documents/HHPGM_FINAL_CH7.PDF

Dinh-Zarr, T. B., Sleet, D. A., Shults, R. A., Zaza, S., Elder, R. W., Nichols, J. L. … Sosin, D. M. (2001). Reviews of evidence regarding interventions to increase the use of safety belts. *American Journal of Preventive Medicine, 21*(4), 48–65.

Goodman, R. M., McLeroy, K. R., Steckler, A. B., & Hoyle, R. H. (1993). Development of level of institutionalization scales for health promotion programs. *Health Education Quarterly, 20*(2), 161–178.

Health Resources and Services Administration (2012). *Dynamics of sustainability.* Department of Health and Human Resources, pp. 1–43. Retrieved from https://www.ruralhealthinfo.org/assets/1211-4984/dynamics-of-sustainability.pdf

Luke, D., Calhoun, A., Robichaux, C., Elliott, M., & Moreland-Russell, S. (2014). The program sustainability assessment tool: A new instrument for public health programs. *Preventing Chronic Disease, 11,* 130184. doi:10.5888/pcd11.130184

Merriam Webster (2018). *Definition of sustainability.* Retrieved from https://www.merriam-webster.com/dictionary/sustainability

Plan-International (2012). *Programme Briefing: Lessons from a post-intervention study in Taita-Taveta District, Kenya. Issue 1:* August 2012, p. 1–4. Retrieved from http://valuingvoices.com/wp-content/uploads/2017/01/PLAN-KENYA-Programme-Briefing-Post-intervention-study-WEB.pdf

Pluye, P., Potvin, L., & Denis, J. L. (2004). Making public health programs last: Conceptualizing sustainability. *Evaluation and Program Planning, 27*(2), 121–133. doi:10.1016/j.evalprogplan.2004.01.001

Scheirer, M. A. (2005). Is sustainability possible? A review and commentary on empirical studies of program sustainability. *American Journal of Evaluation, 26*(3), 320–347. doi:10.1177/1098214005278752

Substance Abuse and Mental Health Services Administration (2013). *Safe schools/healthy students initiative national evaluation: 2005–2008 Cohorts.* Rockville, MD. Retrieved from https://store.samhsa.gov/shin/content/SMA13-4798/SSHS_National_Evaluation.pdf

Substance Abuse and Mental Health Services Administration Center for the Application of Prevention Technologies (2012). *Planning for Sustainability.* Retrieved from http://captus.samhsa.gov/access-resources/planning-sustainability

United States Department of Health and Human Services (2016). *Program Mangers Guide to Evaluation.* Administration for Children and Families Office of Planning, Research, and Evaluation. p. 1. Retrieved from https://www.acf.hhs.gov/sites/default/files/opre/program_managers_guide_to_eval2010.pdf

United States Environmental Protection Agency (2014). *What are some of the challenges facing rural and small town America?* Retrieved from https://www.epa.gov/sites/production/files/2014-06/documents/ref_herman_081612.pdf

Windmoller, M., (2013). *Achieving policy change rural communities.* Community Commons. Retrieved from https://www.communitycommons.org/2013/09/achieving-policy-change-in-rural-communities/

Yin, R. K. (1979). *Changing urban bureaucracies: How new practices become routinized.* Lexington, MA: Lexington Books.

Yin, R. K. (1981). Life histories of innovations: How new practices become routinized. *Public Administration Review, 41,* 21–28.

APPENDIX A

LOGIC MODEL

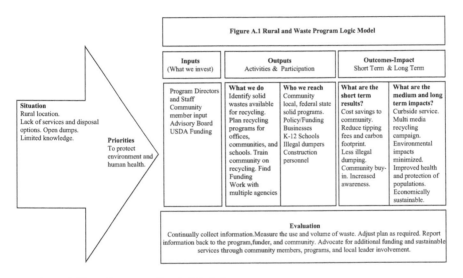

A.1 Rural Waste Program Logic Model.

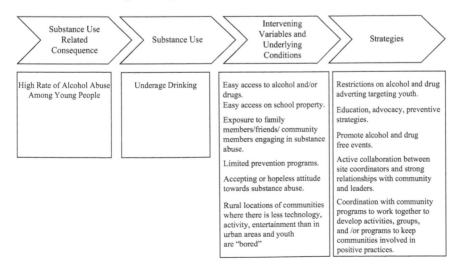

A.2 Intervening Variables Logic Model.

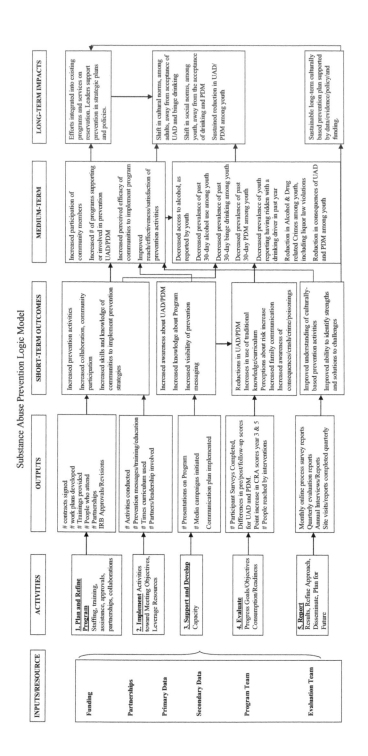

Substance Abuse Prevention Logic Model

A.3 Rural Prevention Program Logic Model.

APPENDIX B

EVALUATION DATA COLLECTION

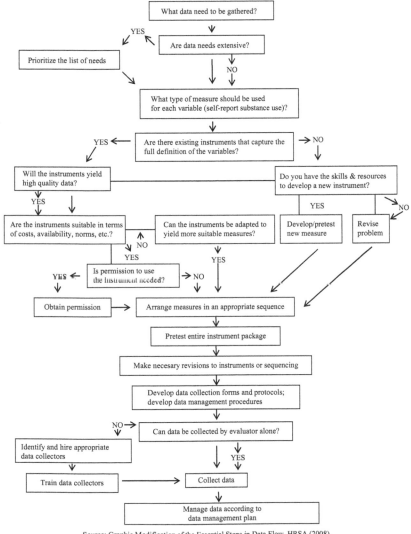

B.1 Data Collection Plan.

APPENDIX C

INSTITUTIONAL REVIEW BOARD

Checklist for ethical evaluation

_____You know what ethics means based on the program and context that you are working in.

_____You understand that ethical behavior is important in rural communities for:

- Program effectiveness
- Standing in the community
- Credibility and leadership
- Professional and legal issues

_____You have decided on the confidentiality level participant's information.

_____You have informed your participants of this.

_____You asked for consent to share information if necessary.

_____You have used disclosure in situations where deemed necessary.

_____The organziation is competent to accomplish its goals under reasonable circumstances.

_____You have taken steps to eliminate conflict situations when they arise.

_____You know how to deal with unethical behavior from individuals and organizations.

_____You know your ethical responsibilities.

_____You keep evaluation procedures as brief as possible, and provide incentives to encourage participation in the evaluation.

Source: Adapted from the Community Tool Box: Section 5 Ethical Isseus in Community Interventions (2018).

Documenting approval of the evaluation plan

In this book, we focused on developing an evaluation plan, but we did not discuss who approves the evaluation plan. The approval of the evaluation plan is largely dependent on the funding agency and evaluation purpose. Below is an example of how a five-year rural program evaluation funded by SAMHSA (Substance Abuse Mental Health Services Administration) was approved.

1. Develop first draft of plan using the five-step process outlined in Chapter 5. By this time all instruments and data sources that will be used to answer the evaluation questions and fulfill the evaluation purpose have been piloted, identified, and established.
2. Document community feedback in evaluation plan, who provided what feedback, and when.
3. Revise evaluation plan and redistribute to community. Submit evaluation plan to the SAMHSA project officer.
4. Wait six months for SAMHSA review. SAMHSA gave evaluation plan to their technical assistance team to review and comment.
5. Receive comments from SAMHSA, revise to include additional measures (prescription drug abuse). Send revised evaluation plan back to SAMHSA.
6. Wait one month for SAMHSA approval. Receive approval. Prepare Institutional Review Board (IRB) application.
7. Identify IRBs of record for the communities involved in the evaluation. Prepare and submit evaluation plan, forms, surveys, rationale, and budget to IRBs.
8. Wait two months for the IRB to review. Respond to reviewer suggestions. Receive written approval from the IRB that the protocol was deemed evaluation and therefore exempt by OHRP standards and IRB members.
9. Program evaluation begins.
10. Provide annual updates to the IRB about the project.

Confidentiality form example

Organization Name Here

Research Confidentiality Agreement for Research Involving Human Participants

I [insert the name of person who is working on project] have agreed to assist with [insert what he or she will be doing] or the research project entitled [title here], IRB# [IRB protocol number].

I agree not to discuss or disclose any of the content or personal information contained within the data, tapes, transcriptions or other research records with anyone other than the Principal Investigator [insert PI's name or name of person listed on the IRB protocol] or in the context of the research team. I agree to maintain confidentiality at all times and abide by the [insert the name of the organization] policies and procedures for ethics in research and the [insert name of organization and title of appropriate policies] on the protection of human subjects in research.

Date:

Signed

Principal Investigator Signature

To be completed by all members of the research or evaluation team with access to person data on human research participations.

File a copy with the PI.

Office of Human Research Protections

The Office for Human Research Protections (OHRP) provides guidance and resources for institutional review boards (IRBs), investigators, and others to determine if an evaluation activity is research involving human subjects. Evaluations must be reviewed by an IRB under the requirements of the US Department of Health and Human Services (HHS) regulations at 45 CFR part 46. In some cases, an evaluation may be reviewed using expedited procedures and in other cases informed consent or documentation may be waived (OHRP, 2016).

Ethical guidelines for program evaluation are often tied to the discipline from which the program originates (e.g. social work). Evaluators are responsible for following guidelines and ensuring that evaluations benefit others, do not harm, are fair, and respect others rights.

Collecting data from individuals requires that evaluators protect confidentiality and act in an ethical manner. Evaluators must let individuals know why they are collecting information, how much time is needed to participate, risk associated with participation, how information will be used and reported, and communicate that results will be confidential.

If evaluators are not collecting personally identifiable information (address, birth date, and social security number), they may not be required to obtain informed consent. If the evaluator is collecting identifiable information, informed consent must be obtained. In some cases, consent is not required (public places and nonformal settings). Participation is always voluntary and individuals should know they can choose not to complete the evaluation.

Special groups

When conducting an evaluation with minors (<18 years), active or passive consent must be sent to the minor's parent or guardian. If children are less than seven years, assent is required. Other vulnerable groups and guidelines can be viewed at www.hhs.gov/ohrp.

Office of Human Research Protections (2016). *Regulations and Policy Decision Charts*. Retrieved from www.hhs.gov/ohrp/regulations-and-policy/decision-charts/index.html

Adult consent form

Date:

Program:

Dear Participant,

My name is [insert your name here] and I am the Evaluator for [insert the program here]. We would like you to participate in an evaluation of [insert here]. The evaluation will ask questions about [insert focus of evaluation questions here]. We will also ask you to complete evaluations of [insert program activities or others here]. Your feedback will be used to [insert how you will use the information].

Your responses will be anonymous. No identifiable information will be collected and no one, including the Lead Evaluator or the [insert program name] will link any information to you. However, the information provided may be used in publications/presentations.

Your consent and participation are completely voluntary. You may withdraw at any time. There is no reward for participating or consequence for not participating. Any risks associated with participation in the evaluation are no greater than those of daily living.

For further information on this evaluation please contact [insert the name of the lead evaluator here, insert phone or email here]. If you have any questions about this evaluation, please contact the [insert program director or agency contact name and number or email here].

There are two copies of this letter. After signing them, keep one copy for your records and return the other during the first [activity, meeting, or event].

"By signing below I agree to allow my child to participate."

Signature: _____

Name (please print): _____

Date: _____

Youth assent form

Date:

Program:

Dear Youth Participant:

My name is [insert evaluator's name here] and I am the Lead Evaluator [insert program name here]. The evaluation will ask questions about your [insert focus of evaluation]. We will also ask you to complete evaluations of various [events, activities, etc.]. Your feedback will be used to [insert how the information will be used].

Taking the evaluation is voluntary. This means you do not have to complete the evaluation if you don't want to. Nothing will happen to you if you decide not to participate.

If you agree to participate you will complete the evaluation using a pen and paper. You will not be able to put your name on the evaluation and your answers will be completely private. We may use some of the information you provide for publications and presentations.

Please read the following and sign below if you agree to participate.

"I understand that:

• if I don't want to take the evaluation that's ok and I won't get into trouble
• anytime that I want to stop participating that's ok
• my name will not be known and my answers will be completely private
• any risks in the study are no greater than those of daily living"

For further information on this evaluation please contact [insert the name of the lead evaluator here, insert phone or email here]. If you have any questions about this evaluation, please contact the [insert program director or agency contact name and number or email here].

There are two copies of this letter. After signing each copy, keep one copy for your records. Bring the second signed copy with you to the first [meeting, event, program].

Signature: _____

Name (please print): _____

Date: _____

Photo release form for children/youth

[for adult release form simply modify the language]

I agree that [insert program name here] may photograph and record my child/dependent's likeness and activities (Images) during the program. I grant the following rights to [insert program name]: permission to use and reuse, publish and republish, and modify or alter the Image(s) taken during the shoot. Use of the Images for editorial, commercial, trade, advertising, and any other purpose may be done in any medium now existing or subsequently developed, on the [program website] and on the Internet, and worldwide in perpetuity for the purposes stated above.

I waive my right to inspect or approve any editorial text or copy that is used in connection with the images and release and discharge [program name] from any and all claims arising out of use of the images for the purposes described above, including any claims for libel, invasion of privacy, or another tortuous act.

I have read the foregoing. I fully understand its contents, understand that this agreement does not expire, and confirm my agreement by signing below. I am over the age of 21 and have legal capacity to sign the release.

Child/Youth's Name (print)	Parent/Guardian Name (print)
X	X
Parent/Guardian Signature	Date
Street Address	City, State, Zip
Parent/Guardian Email	Phone

APPENDIX D

FORMS AND EXAMPLES

Six month evaluation timeline and tasks example

Tasks	Month 1	Month 2	Month 3	Month 4	Month 5	Month 6
Finalize contract	X					
Obtain and review prior grant reports, data.	X	X				
Obtain input on evaluation approach, data, tools, and forms	X	X	X			
Quarterly meeting [etc.]		X	X		X	X
Finalize evaluation plan and submit IRB application		X	X			
Recruit and retain evaluation associates			X			
Data coordination	X		X			
Surveys, interviews, site specific evaluation	X		X			
Community site visits		X		X		X
Evaluation training available		X	X			
Data collection and Analysis	X	X	X			
Monthly online process evaluations	X	X	X	X	X	X
Data reporting				X	X	X
Technical assistance available	X	X	X	X	X	X

Program budget example

Budget category	Justification	Rate and Level of effort	Total charged to program
Personnel	Project director/name	$60,000 and 10%	$6,000.00
Fringe	Retirement 10%, FICA 7.65%, Insurance 6%, Social security 6%	29.65%	$1,779.00
Travel	Mandatory program meeting Project director	Airfare—$200/Flight Hotel—$180/2 nights Per Diem—$46 per day × 2 days	$652.00
Equipment	Copy machine	1 @ $5,200 and 100% charged to program	$5,200.00
Supplies	Laptop computer	1 @ $900.00	$900.00
Contracts	Evaluator	$40 per hour × 225 hours for 12 months	$9,000.00
Construction	Not authorized under this program		
Other	Rent	$15/sq. × 700 sq. feet	$10,500.00
Total direct costs	$34,031.00		
Indirect costs	Fixed IDC rate	8%	$2,722.48
Total program costs	$36,753.48		

Event cover sheet example

Title of Event _____ Date(s) _____ Location _____

Funding Amount _____ Number of Individuals Reached _____ (attach sign-in sheet)

Data Collected ___ Yes (if yes, list data collection instruments below) ___ No

Purpose: [insert purpose of event]

_____

_____

List primary programs involved in funding and/or planning this activity:

_____

_____

_____

Target Population (circle all that apply)
[Insert target populations that may be represented]

Did this event accomplish your purpose? Please describe.

_____

_____

_____

_____

Select Program Goals this activity supports (select all that apply):
_____ [Insert program goals here]
Select Objectives this activity supports from the list below (select all that apply):
_____ [Insert program objectives here]
Other Notes

_____
_____
_____

Protocol for administering survey example

Project title:

Instrument/survey title:

What is being measured:

Target audience:

How to collect information:

[This survey was developed to.... Individuals will have identified from sign-in sheets and eligibility will be confirmed prior to gaining consent/assent of participant]
Where to obtain copies of this tool:

Things to note before using this survey:

Languages available:

Understanding before and after example

[if desired, include questions on age, gender, community, or program here]

1. Circle your level of understanding of [insert topic or focus] before and after the event.

Before

1   2   3   4   5
Basic Understanding   Advance Understanding

After

1   2   3   4   5
Basic Understanding   Advance Understanding
[Add as many before and after statements as needed].

2.   Rate your level of satisfaction of the event, 1 is low satisfaction and 5 is high satisfaction.

LOW   HIGH
1   2   3   4   5

3.   From the list below, select two statements that best describe how the event impacted you. If you were not impacted leave this section blank.

_____I feel more [insert here]

_____I have increased knowledge about [insert information here]

_____I have new skills to [insert information here]

_____I have increased knowledge about [insert information here]

_____I have increased confidence in [insert information here]

_____Other, please describe_____

Activity feedback form example

Q1 What is your zip code? _____
[include other demographic as appropriate, use gender neutral questions when asking about gender]
Q2 How did you learn about this event?

O   Website_____
O   Flyer
O   Email
O   Friend
O   Driving by event location
O   Work

Other_____
Q3 Why did you come to the event?

_____

Rate the following [etc.]	*Importance of Topic* *1=Not Important* *5=Very Important*	*Likelihood That You* *Will Use Information* *1= Not at All Likely* *5= Very Likely*
Workforce challenges—Dr. Johnson	1 2 3 4 5	1 2 3 4 5
[etc.]	1 2 3 4 5	1 2 3 4 5
[etc.]	1 2 3 4 5	1 2 3 4 5

Key informant interview guide example

Name: _____ Day: _____
Affiliation: _____ Start/End Time: _____
Position: _____ Verbal Consent: _____

Hi, my name is [insert name] and I am working with [program name] to learn more about [insert the focus or rationale]. Our interview will take about [average time based on pilot testing], are you willing to be interviewed? Do you have any questions before we begin?

1. Tell me about your experience with [etc.]
2. What are some of the strengths [etc.]?
3. What are some challenges [etc.]
4. What needs to happen to [etc.]
   Probe: Think back to the challenges we talked about in #3. What could be done about those?)
5. What components are essential for [etc.]
6. Do you have any other thoughts or opinions that should be considered for [etc.]?

Needs of community example

Figure D.1 may be used in communities during the needs assessment process or in developing priorities for the program or evaluation. Using photos or drawings to focus the discussion and data collection effort may be helpful. This method, visual participatory data collection, was used by a rural community to

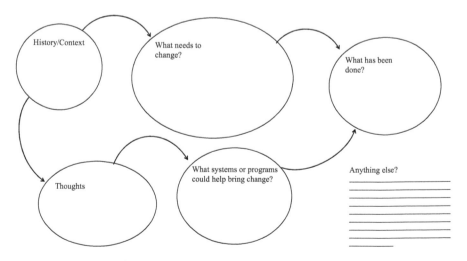

FIGURE D.1 Needs of Community.

discuss mental health and substance use needs after focus groups and traditional surveys did not work.

Evaluation report outline example

1. Background

    a. Evaluation Approach
    b. Data Sources and Methods

2. Staff Development and Staff Training Activities
3. Program Goals

    a. Community Readiness to Support Program Goals 2 and 3
    b. Activities that Decrease Program Focus Goal 4
    c. Individual Program Services, Goal 1

4. Documenting the Impact of the Program
5. Process Evaluation Summary

    a. Success
    b. Challenges

6. Outcome Evaluation Summary
7. Limitations
8. Conclusion
9. Appendix A Training Agendas
10. Appendix B Team Member Bios
11. Appendix C Partners and Programs
12. Appendix D Main Findings Short Report
13. Appendix E Budget Summary

INDEX

acculturation 28
accuracy 36
accurate information 103; *see also* information
active listening strategies 74
administrative data 86, 97–8
Adobe InDesign 136
adversary-oriented evaluation 46
African Americans 14, 17, 36, 39, 108
African Evaluation Association (AfrEA) 36–7
Alaska Native 21–2
alternative intervention 58
American Evaluation Association (AEA) 3, 28, 31, 158–9
American Evaluation Association Cultural Competence in Evaluation Task Force 31
American Indian Higher Education Consortium 38
American Indian populations 21, 40
American Public Health Association 158
American Revolution 2
analysis of variance (ANOVA) 107–8
analytic horizon 57
analytic methods 110
arthritis campaign in rural Arkansas 152
assessment 126–7
audience 57, 142

Bailey, Sandra 40
Ball, T.J. 38
basic research 63

bike/pedestrian trails 128–9
budget and program costs 76–8
Bureau of Labour and Statistics 16

categories 110
Centers for Disease Control and Prevention 37, 134, 163, 164–5
channels 142
child poverty 17
Chi-square tests 107
Clama, Katherine 32
cluster evaluation 48
coding 110
community(ies): culture and 27; defined 2; needs of 78; in rural America 13; three types of 13
Community-Based Participatory Research (CBPR) 38
community concerns 78
community members 71–4
comparison groups 58
competence: rural evaluators 31; *see also specific entries*
constructivist paradigm 4
consumer-oriented evaluation 46
construct validity 109
content analysis 110
content validity 95
context: defined 11, 28; field notes on 12; and place 11–12
Context Income Reaction and Outcome (CIRO) evaluation 47
continuous data 98

convergent parallel designs 62
Corporation for National and Community
  Service (CNCS) 156
correlation analyses 108
cost analysis 58
cost–benefit analysis 58
cost-effectiveness analysis 58
costs: fixed 58; variable 58
cost of rural evaluation 156
cost utility 58
Council for State and Territorial
  Epidemiologists 158
Cramer, Katherine 20
credibility: establishing 73
cross-cultural, defined 28
cultural competence 27–41; African
  Evaluation Association (AfrEA)
  guidelines 36–7; case examples with
  specific cultures in rural America 39–40;
  changing culture 32–4; Culturally and
  Linguistically Appropriate Services
  standards 35; culturally competent
  resources 37–8; culture 27–8; defined
  28; examples of standards supporting
  35–7; guiding principles for rural
  evaluators 31–2; Joint Committee on
  Standards for Educational Evaluation
  36; national education association 35–6;
  rural communities and 29–30; seeking
  involvement 30; tools for assessing an
  evaluator's 34–5
culturally competent evaluation: checklist
  for culturally appropriate evaluation
  methods 34; field notes on 33; guiding
  principles for 33; participatory
  approaches supporting 38
culturally competent evaluators 33–4
culturally competent resources 37–8
Culturally Responsive Assessment Tool 35
Culturally Responsive Evaluation 4
Culturally Responsive Evaluation and
  Assessment (CREA) Resource
  Center 37
cultural responsiveness 28
culture 27–8; changing 32–4; community
  and 27; defined 19; dominant 28; field
  notes on 30; group factors 27; individual
  factors 27; of rural America 32; of urban
  areas 32

data: administrative 86, 97–8; amount of
  95; assumptions from 114; collection of
  85, 94–5; continuous 98; defined 105;
  descriptive 107; discrete 98; extant 86;

inferential 107; interval 104; learnings
  from 114; limitations from 114; nominal
  104; ordinal 104; preparing 104;
  presenting 135–6; primary 86, 97–8;
  qualitative 93–4; quantitative 93–4; ratio
  104; scale 104; secondary 86, 97–8; small
  sample size 85–6; types of 93; see also
  specific entries
data agreements 85
data analysis 104–5; assumptions from the
  data 114; grounded theory 109; learnings
  from the data 114; limitations from the
  data 114; mixed methods 113; qualitative
  109–12; quantitative 105–8; quantitative
  validity and reliability 108–9; software
  114; thematic 111–12
data analysis plan 104
data collection B.1; credible evidence 96–7;
  data quality 103–4; data sources 97–8;
  develop and pilot evaluation instruments
  95–6; funding agency reports and grant
  proposals 100–1; news and Internet
  101–2; observations 101; preparing
  the data 104; process 93–7; qualitative
  methods of 99–100; quantitative methods
  of 98–9; review results and refine process
  96; using various data sources 97
data collection methods: qualitative 99–100;
  quantitative 98–9
data collection plan 83–7
data collection strategy 84
data management 85
data ownership 85
data quality 103–4; instrumentation factors
  related to 103; measurement factors
  related to 103; programmatic 103
data sources 97–8; primary data 97–8;
  secondary data 97–8
deaths, and rural America 14
Denver Post 20
Department of Housing Urban
  Development 164
depopulation: defined 14; and rural
  America 14
descriptive data 107
digital storytelling 100
discourse analysis 110
discrete data 98
diversity: defined 14; rural America 14
dominant culture 28

economic evaluation 56–8, 127–9;
  considerations for 57; formulas for
  calculating 58

Economic Research Service 17
economy: rural America 16–17
education 2, 13–14, 18, 21
education associations 158–9
employment: rural America 16–17
empowerment evaluation 4, 48–9
Environmental Protection Agency 158
Ethnic-Sensitive Inventory 35
European Union 157
evaluability assessment 48
evaluand 3
evaluation 3–4; and accountability standards
    36; American Evaluation Association's
    definition of 3; cultural competence
    in 27–41; defined 3; research and
    63–5; resources available for 76–8;
    rural context-focused 22; utilizing
    for policy change and community
    transformation 170
evaluation budgets 76
evaluation design 61–2; field notes on, in
    rural practice 63
evaluation findings: recommendations for
    applying 142–3
evaluation findings, reporting 133–5;
    clarity and purpose 135; defining target
    audience or recipients 134; dissemination
    plan 134–5; engaging stakeholders
    133–4; evaluation report 135
evaluation instruments 95–6
evaluation model: defined 59; logic models
    59–61; outcome sequence chart 61
evaluation plan: conceptual framework 82;
    designing 80–2; goals and objectives in
    74–6
evaluation report: background 137; basic
    elements of 136–41; evaluation purpose
    137–8; executive summary 136–7;
    key findings 139–40; methods 138–9;
    recommendations and lessons learned
    140–1
evaluation research 63, 64
evaluation results: best practices for
    disseminating 143–6; communicating
    141–2
evaluators: culturally competent 33–4;
    develop evaluation goals with
    community participation 75; role 6
"Evaluation use: Advances, challenges, and
    applications" (Leviton) 151
Evergreen, Stephanie 135
executive summary 136–7
experimental designs 61
expertise-oriented evaluation 46

explanatory sequential designs 62
exploratory sequential designs 62
extant data 86
external validity 95, 109

feasibility 36
Federal Office of Rural Health Policy
    (FORHP) 1–2
Federal Register 6
Fisher, P.A. 38
fixed costs 58
focus groups 100
formal evaluation 49
formative evaluation 120–1; defined 52
forms and examples 184–9
funding: rural solicitation for 6
funding agency reports and grant proposals
    100–1

Gardner, Cory 20
goals: defined 74; in the evaluation plan
    74–5; SMART 75
Goldsmith, Harold 2
Goldsmith Method 2
Great Depression 2
Great Recession 16
Great Society Legislation 120
grounded theory data analysis 109

Hazlett, Anne 102
health: rural America 14–16
health care 18
Health Resources Services Administration
    (HRSA) 167
Healthy Schools/Healthy Students
    initiative 167
Hispanic 14, 17, 32, 39, 108, 126–7
honesty, of rural evaluators 31
Hood, Rodney 36
hypotheses testing 107

Idaho Consortium for Safe Schools Healthy
    Students 39
impact evaluation 124–6; defined 53; five
    criteria for 54; formula 53; impact
    indicators 54; indicators 54; measures
    54; monitoring 54; outcome evaluation
    54, 55; principles of 54; targets and
    benchmarks 54
impact indicators 54
indicators 54
Indigenous Evaluation Framework (IEF) 38
Indigenous Focused Evaluation 4
inductive analysis 109

industrialization 2
inferential data 107
informal evaluation 49
information: accurate 103; reliable 103
"In search of impact: An analysis of the
    utilization of federal health evaluation
    research" (Patton) 151
Institutional Review Board (IRB) 87,
    178–83
instrument reliability 95
instrument validity 95
integrity, of rural evaluators 31
intermediate outcomes 55
internal validity 109
Internet 101–2
interval data 104
interviews: defined 99; semistructured 99;
    structured 99; unstructured 99

Joint Committee on Standards for
    Educational Evaluation 36

Kentucky Homeplace 128
Kirkpatrick's evaluation approach 47

language 29
Letiecq, Bethany 40
Licther, Daniel 14
Lincoln, Yvonna 4
linguistic competence 28
listening 74
logic models 59–61, A.2–A.3
long-term outcomes 55
Lucid Press 136

management-oriented evaluation 46
mean 107
measures 54
Medicare 15
Mertens, Donna 20
messages 141
Microsoft Smart Art 60–1
Microsoft Word 136
*Mixed Methods and Credibility of Evidence in
    Evaluation* (Mertens and Hesse-Biber) 73
mixed methods data analysis 113
mixed-methods designs 62
mixed-methods validity 113
monitoring 54
monitoring evaluation (ME) 47
multiculturalism 28
multicultural populations 39

National Center for Cultural Competence
    at Georgetown University 38

National Education Association 35–6
National Rural Health Association 16
National Science Foundation (NSF) 37;
    Beyond Rigor website 37
National Standards for Culturally and
    Linguistically Appropriate Services
    (CLAS) in Health and Health Care 35
Native American 14, 21, 32, 39
Native American Caucus of the California
    Democratic Party 21
natural resources 18
news 101–2
nominal data 104
nonexperimental designs 61
notice of award (NOA) 6
Notice of Solicitation of Applications
    (NOSA) 6

Obama, Barack 17
objectives of analysis 57
objectives-based impact evaluation 48
objectives-oriented evaluation 46
Office of Management and Budget (OMB)
    1–2
older adults 39–40
ordinal data 104
outcome evaluations 54, 123–4; impact
    evaluation and 55; reasons for 55
outcome sequence chart 61
outcomes: intermediate 55; long-term 55;
    short-term 55

paradigm 4–5; constructivist 4; defined 4;
    transformative 4
parameter, defined 105
participant-oriented evaluation 47
participatory/collaborative evaluation 48
Participatory Culture-Specific Consultation
    (PCSC) 38
Participatory Rural Appraisal (PRA) 48
Patton, Michael Quinn 49, 63, 151
performance assessment 56; process
    questions in 56
performance measures and outcomes 87–8
performance monitoring 55–6; defined 52
persistent poverty 17
Pew Research Center 20
phenomenology 110
Phillips's evaluation approach 47
Pictochart 136
policy, defined 170
policy evaluations 170
political context in rural America 19–22
Politics of Resentment (Cramer) 20
population: defined 105

posttest-only design 83
poverty: child 17; persistent 17; in rural
    America 17
power 29
Presenting Data Effectively (Evergreen) 135
Preservation Alliance of West Virginia
    (PAWV) 155–6
pretest/posttest design 83
primary data 86, 97–8
probability sampling 99
process evaluation 122–3; defined 52;
    designing 52
professional associations 158–9
program, defined 46
program evaluation approaches 45–7,
    64; adversary-oriented evaluation
    46; consumer-oriented evaluation
    46; Context Income Reaction and
    Outcome (CIRO) evaluation 47;
    expertise-oriented evaluation 46;
    Kirkpatrick's evaluation approach 47;
    management-oriented evaluation 46;
    objectives-oriented evaluation 46;
    participant-oriented evaluation 47;
    Phillips's evaluation approach 47; Success
    Case Method (SCM) 47
programmatic data quality 103
Program Sustainability Assessment Tool
    (PSAT) 165
Project Excellence in Partnerships for
    Community Outreach, Research and
    Training (EXPORT) 126–7
propriety 36
public welfare 32
published literature: challenges from 151–3;
    rural evaluators and 151–3
Publisher 136

qualitative data 93–4
qualitative data analysis 109–12; coding 110;
    discourse analysis 110; grounded theory
    data analysis 109; inductive analysis
    109; phenomenology 110; qualitative
    approaches 109–12; qualitative validity
    112; thematic data analysis 111–12
qualitative data collection methods 99–100
qualitative validity 112
quantitative data 93–4, 105–8; analyzing
    105–9; collection methods 98–9
quantitative reliability 108–9
quantitative validity 108–9
quasi-experimental designs 61

random sample 105
Rapid Rural Appraisal (RRA) 48

ratio data 104
real-world evaluation 4
reliability: instrument 95; quantitative
    108–9
reliable information 103; *see also*
    information
research: basic 63; defined 63; and
    evaluation 63–5
resources available for evaluation 76–8
respect 72–3
routinization 166
rural America: case examples with specific
    cultures in 39–40; characteristics of 13–14;
    deaths in 14; depopulation in 14; diversity
    in 14; education in 18; employment and
    economy 16–17; health care and 18; health
    disparities in 14–16; living in 13; natural
    resources 18; political context in 19–22;
    poverty in 17; rural context-focused
    evaluation 22; rural populations 14; social
    context of 19; technology and 18; three
    types of communities in 13
rural citizen engagement plan 153
rural head start classrooms 123–4
rural communities 1–3; cultural
    competence and 29–30; evaluation
    approaches frequently used in 47–9
rural community evaluation: characteristics
    of rural America 12–14; context and
    place 11–12; defined 4; employment
    and economy 16–17; health disparities
    14–16; poverty 17; technology, health
    care, education, and natural resources
    17–22
rural community evaluation process:
    building trust 72; community concerns
    78; community needs 78; data collection
    plan 83–7; designing the evaluation
    plan 80–2; engaging stakeholders and
    community members 71–4; establish
    credibility 73; goals and objectives
    in evaluation plan 74–6; Institutional
    Review Board (IRB) 87; listening 74;
    performance measures and outcomes
    87–8; plan for sharing results 88;
    planning 70–1; resources available for the
    evaluation 76–8; respect 72–3; theories
    82–3; time lines 83; work plan 79–80
rural consciousness 20
rural context-focused evaluation 22
rural evaluation 4; process of 5–6; selecting the
    right approach for 65; text dedicated to 5
rural evaluators: arthritis campaign in rural
    Arkansas 152; balancing program needs
    with funding agency requirements 150;

challenges from published literature 151–3; challenges from the field 149–51; competence 31; cost of rural evaluation 156; education and professional associations 158–9; fitting well with community and evaluation 153–4; guiding principles for 31–2; hiring an evaluator, contracts and agreements 154–6; honesty and integrity 31; limited resources and staffing 150–1; local policies and staffing 150; opportunities for 157–8; other cost considerations 156–7; preparation and education 150; process evaluation challenges 152; program theories fail to explain outcomes 151; respect for people 31–2; responsibilities for general and public welfare 32; rural health department evaluation 152; school-based behavioral health program evaluation 151; slow to change 151; social change 157; statement of work (SOW) 149; systematic inquiry 31; workforce development 158
rural health department evaluation 152
Rural Health Information Hub 78
rural Hispanic populations 39
rural populations 2, 4, 14, 22, 143
rural programs: implementing 6–7; planning 6–7; sustaining 6–7
rural solicitation for funding 6

sample: defined 105; random 105
scale data 104
Scheirer, Mary Ann 167
school-based behavioral health program evaluation 151
secondary data 86, 97–8
semistructured interviews 99
short-term outcomes 55
SMART goals 75, 89
social change: rural evaluators 157
social context of rural America 19
social planning 170
software 114
sources 142
stakeholders 71–4
standard deviation 107
statement of work (SOW) 149
statistical significance 107
statistics: defined 105
structured interviews 99
Substance Abuse and Mental Health Services Administration (SAMHSA) 59, 163
Success Case Method (SCM) 47

surveys 98–9
sustainability: defining 163–4; evaluation methods focusing on 168–9; factors influencing 167–8; funding future work on 169; sustained impacts 168; utilizing evaluation for policy change and community transformation 170
sustainability plan 165–6
Sustained Emerging Impacts Evaluation (SEIE) 168–9
sustained impacts: evaluation methods focusing on 168–9
Swidler, Ann 19
systematic inquiry 31

target population 58
targets and benchmarks 54
technology 18
thematic data analysis 111–12
themes 110
theories 82–3
theory-driven evaluation 49
Three Approaches to Qualitative Content Analysis Content (Hsieh and Shannon) 110
time, defined 94
time lines 83
time-series design 83
transformative paradigms 4
tribal governments 21
Tribal Participatory Research (TPR) 38
Tribal Participatory Research Model 38
Trump, Donald 20
trust building 72
t-tests 107
Tyler, Ralph 46

United States Census Bureau 1
United States Department of Agriculture Economic Research Service 86
United States Department of Agriculture (USDA) 13, 76, 102
United States Department of Health and Human Services 158
United States Department of Health and Human Services (USDHHS) Office of Minority Health 35
unstructured interviews 99
urbanization 2
US Agency for International Development (USAID) 157
US Department of Agriculture Children Youth and Families At-Risk grant 40
US Department of Education: Student Mentoring Program 125–6

US Department of Health and Human Services Office of Human Research Protections 87
utility 36
utilization-focused evaluation (UFE) 4, 48–9

Validity 28; construct 109; content 95; external 95, 109; instrument 95; internal 109; mixed-methods 113; qualitative 112; quantitative 108–9
variable costs 58
variable, defined 106

variance 107
viewpoints 57

Washington Post-Kaiser Family Foundation 19
Weber, Max 166
Western cultures 31
W.K. Kellogg Foundation 48
workforce development 158
work plan 79–80
World Health Organization 157
World War II 2

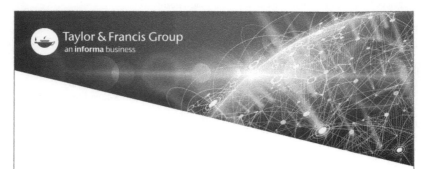

Milton Keynes UK
Ingram Content Group UK Ltd.
UKHW031149141024
449569UK00024B/945